THE EFFICIENT PORT

THE EFFICIENT PORT

R. B. ORAM

AND

C. C. R. BAKER

PERGAMON PRESS

Oxford · New York · Toronto
Sydney · Braunschweig

Pergamon Press Ltd., Headington Hill Hall, Oxford

Pergamon Press Inc., Maxwell House, Fairview Park, Elmsford,
New York 10523

Pergamon of Canada Ltd., 207 Queen's Quay West, Toronto 1

Pergamon Press (Aust.) Pty. Ltd., 19a Boundary Street,
Rushcutters Bay, N.S.W. 2011, Australia

Vieweg & Sohn GmbH, Burgplatz 1, Braunschweig

First edition 1971
Library of Congress Catalog Card No. 78–135098

Printed in Great Britain by A. Wheaton & Co., Exeter

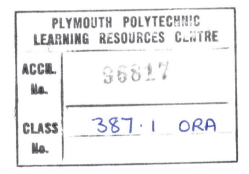
08 016396 3

CONTENTS

v

INTRODUCTION

In *The Efficient Port* the authors have tried to set out conditions as they are in the major ports of the world at the time of writing. They are aware that the port and shipping industry, after many years of near stagnation, has developed so rapidly since 1945 that a mere record of the changes that have been telescoped into the last quarter of a century would in itself be a major operation. In attempting this, they have, for the benefit of the overwhelming number of smaller ports overseas, brought in suggestions for the improvement of cargo handling; these are based on their lifetime's experience of the industry.

The authors have tried to give this book, which is a successor to *Cargo Handling and the Modern Port*, published in this series in 1965, an international appeal, and they hope that it will be a help to the many port authorities and others whose vital interest is shown by their competition for places, both at the United Nations School of Ports and Shipping, based on Copenhagen, and the International Seminar on Port Management held annually at Delft, Holland. At the same time, attention has been focused on British ports, particularly London, where progress over the last decade has been spectacular.

In the final chapters an attempt has been made, by assembling the latest thinking on the port of the future, to predict the shape and the size that it will take. The authors are certainly aware that it is not within their power to paint a detailed picture of the shape of things to come; some of the forecasts that have been made smack too much of science fiction to be taken seriously; others ignore the human element to an extent that brands them as unrealistic. They feel, however, that it will be at least a decade before the port of the future has settled down into a shape that embodies all the revolutionary changes of the present.

Opportunity has been taken in checking proofs to insert notes of the most recent developments as "Additional Notes", at the end of each chapter.

CHAPTER 1

THE PORT—ITS PRESENT FUNCTIONS

Introduction

At no time in the history of port development have the signs for the practical man been so difficult to read. What is happening to ports all over the world? Is there an accepted shape that the port of the future can be relied upon to take? The Industrial Revolution of the eighteenth century fixed the pattern of ports for the first half of the twentieth century. Save for the gradual changes that followed from sail to steam, the port industry was so near to being static that a Rip van Winkle could, in 1930, have picked up the same handtruck that his grandfather had dropped and over the same cobble stones have trundled similar bales of wool. After 1945 many of the factors that had made for stability disappeared. The very pattern of quays, sheds, and warehouses with which the world of transportation had grown up, was shattered overnight. The familiar background to cargo handling fell apart. The emphasis was henceforth to be on new equipment which made possible new methods of transferring cargo to and from ships and from place to place within the ports. The ancient and primitive science by which legions of dockworkers picked up and put down again millions of man-handled packages gave way to mechanized methods dedicated to the evolution of the largest practical cargo unit. Trends in port working during the last two decades have had one major aim—the substitution of a few dockers working sophisticated machines for gangs of dockers with hand equipment. Apart from those bulk cargoes which have replaced general homogeneous goods, the ultimate unit for mixed cargoes has become the container.

Today every port in the world could truly be said to be involved in the container revolution. At one end of the scale is the small port that sees a possible future only as a small feeder port. At the other is the recently constructed terminal already 100 per cent committed to containers. Between the two extremes lie the majority of ports all over the world

1

which, while they hope to be included in the final pattern of unit transport, are resigned to struggling on with the present admittedly unsatisfactory ways by which cargo is discharged and loaded.

Ports and their problems have always been recognized as being complex. No one man has ever come up with a solution that would treble output overnight. Whether the successful administration of the modern container port will take the port area out of the controversial zone and will reduce it to the smooth running of a factory, is still too soon to predict. It is certain, however, that quite a large proportion of the working areas of the major ports will continue to be faced with problems of efficient working that will keep their owners busy for another decade.

Port authorities and shipping companies in the most highly developed of the maritime nations are now very conscious of the need for improvement in ship turnround. Gone are the days when handling methods were guarded with the security that King Henry the Navigator ensured for the records of his voyages down the African coast. Good cargo handling is seen as the principal factor that will drive out bad. The benefit gained from a speedy turnround in Liverpool is wasted if there is delay through inefficient handling in Bombay. Despite the phenomenal progress made in a few ports with the handling of unit loads and bulk cargo, it is the confident hope of the authors of this book that most world ports will find therein suggestions that will push up their tonnage per man hour—the ultimate criterion of port efficiency.

Ship Turnround

No single cause more directly affects the cost of living of a maritime country than the speed with which ships are turned round in her ports. More than half of the price of an imported article is made up of costs of the transportation that has linked the producer with the consumer. At no point in this chain can costs so easily get out of control as at the port—the vital link that enables sea-going traffic to be transferred to road or rail: this is the primary function of all ports, whatever their shape or size. The speed at which this physical transfer takes place is the criterion of the port's efficiency.

In 1966 the world's total of cargo-carrying tonnage of vessels of 100 gross registered tonnage (g.r.t.) and upwards, amounted to 182,000,000 dead weight tonnage (d.w.t.). The ports in which ships were loaded and discharged covered giants such as Rotterdam and London, and extended down to the few privately owned and shallow-draughted ports giving employment to a few local dockers. There are some 2000 ports in the world of which 200 can handle over a million tons of goods each year.

With the possible exception of a few container ports that can still be counted on the fingers of two hands, none of the many ports that minister to their country's commercial needs are run efficiently. This is an admission that no port authority—whether national, municipal, corporative, or private—will contest. No other industry would so willingly admit such a degree of inefficiency; whilst deploring the causes it is almost helpless to cure them. To list some of the requisites of an efficient port is to illustrate how far most ports are from possessing them. The first requirement is a steady flow of traffic—import, export, and for warehousing—and which would arrive and could be worked independently of weather. Then, a happy band of dockworkers pledged to the good working of the port; sufficient craft, rail wagons, and roads to render the traffic of the port fluid at all times. Lastly, and the most impossible to achieve, a shift system that would make possible a 24-hour working day on each berth for 7 days a week, backed up by an organization that could avoid congestion. With this would go the ability to make up each set lifted to the safe working load of the quay crane or the ship's derricks. In short, in the efficient port work would go on day and night with all the equipment employed to its full capacity. Except for the highly organized work of a few container ports, so desirable a state of affairs has not yet been achieved in practice. For this the port authority is by no means to blame. Most port operators have had to live with the handicap of an inherited estate that perpetuates the designs of their predecessors who, thinking to build for eternity, succeeded only in making posterity their prisoners. The contributory causes to port inefficiency (although the port authority, being on the spot, attracts most of the censure when ports become congested), cover the shipper and the receiver of the cargo, the designer of the ship, the systems of employment of staff and labour, the port engineer, the design and the number of craft, as well as the road and rail layout. In succeeding chapters each of these causes, together with others, will be considered, and remedies that have been found to be effective will be examined. When inefficiency, or port congestion which is the obvious manifestation of this, has drifted into being the accepted conditions of working, then less obvious causes have to be looked for. These may have existed for so long in the history of a particular port that they have formed part pattern of the work there.

Function of the Port

Basically the port does only one thing although it may do this superbly well; it may also do it in a myriad different ways. Unlike a factory a port has no end product—it provides services and facilities for ship turnround. In short, it picks up and puts down again millions of single packages. Each picking up and each putting down advances the cargo unit one stage on its journey from the factory to the shop counter or as part of its transfer from raw material to finished article. To say that a piece of cut timber is handled twelve times between the saw mill in a Baltic village and the house in a London suburb is probably an understatement. It follows, therefore, that port congestion comes about when the number of cargo units to be picked up and put down again is more than the labour available can handle during the time that it is prepared to work. None of the causes of slow turnround to ships in port can get far away from this basic principle.

Some ports have been run on the lines that facilities should not be provided until there is a proven demand for them. This was the guiding light throughout the Victorian era of port development, and it blighted progress until the Second World War swept away many of the old-fashioned buildings that cluttered west European ports. Now the system of providing alternative types of berths so that the prospective user can choose the one that will suit his project the best has been adopted in go-ahead ports such as London and the Benelux terminals.[1]

The Custom of the Port

Parallel with this leap forward has been the growing awareness that a most insidious (because hitherto largely unrecognized) cause of slow turnround is "the custom of the port". This shows itself in many forms and these vary from port to port. All are exceptionally difficult to eradicate because all have been woven into the pattern of the port in forms that suited powerful interests. A custom of the port has been defined as a practice that operates but for which written authority does not exist; therefore it cannot be cancelled. The total of such customs that control work in any port can be formidable. Although the port authority can see the extent to which its efforts at improvement are hamstrung, it is powerless

[1] "By creating the facilities in advance of demand a demand has been created."

to eradicate any of them overnight. Many practical examples come to mind.

Grain discharge made from a bulk-carrying vessel may be demanded for delivery in bags, reducing output from a modern silo to about 1000 tons per day. A portable elevator, used by the receiver to do his own bagging, would enable the silo to work to capacity, making room for an incoming ship. Countries that export cut timber, both hardwood and softwood, impose a dire burden on their ports by tendering cargo in loose pieces. One unit of packaged timber can contain 100 or more pieces and requires only one lift. Similarly, sugar exported in bags is likely to have a limit imposed by quay cranes or ship's gear of 4000 tons on a berth working two shifts a day. A ship that takes sugar on board in bulk can sail within hours of berthing. Plywood is often tendered in single bundles. Units of like size and quality could be strapped together in sets that weighed a ton or more. Similarly, bananas, if the merchantable hands are put into ventilated cartons and these are palletized, can be loaded at a much faster

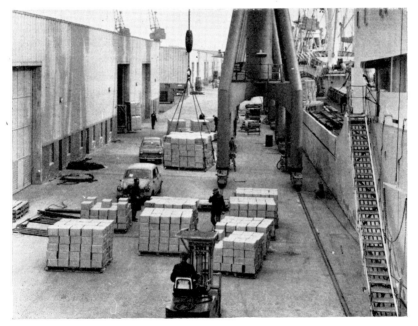

Fig. 1. Palletized export traffic, Tilbury Dock , London. (By courtesy of PLA.)

rate than in single baskets or naked stems and without the damage that is associated with this traffic (Fig. 1). In the past, port authorities have sought to attract traffic by the offer of sorting to marks and grades, thus putting their transit sheds at the disposal of the importer. Fresh fruit thus processed is ready for the market as it leaves the docks. Unfortunately, excessive marking, or merely illegible or insufficient symbols, damaged boxes, or the need for sampling, can and does delay the movement of the goods through the transit shed. Heavy and awkward packages often form part of a ship's cargo. These are often left on the quay to the blockage of through traffic in order to avoid double handling. Poor road access, unsuitable type wagons for bulk cargo or indifferent rail marshalling facilities, a chronic shortage of craft or lack of an internal lighterage system, can all be classed as port customs against which port authorities struggle not always successfully. To end this catalogue of accepted handicaps, the too meticulous conduct of the national Customs can throttle the passage of goods through a port as those who have done business in some eastern ports can bear witness.

Multiple Employers of Port Workers

The decasualization of labour in United Kingdom ports that took place on 18 September 1967 was preceded by a reduction in the number of port employers. A few years ago this stood in the United Kingdom's National Dock Labour Board's Register at about 1400. For all of these to have been effective would have made the general picture of our ports more absurd than it actually was. The various port authorities employed a very high proportion of dock labour, and they were followed by a few major private stevedores. Most of the 1400 were small employers who discharged or loaded an occasional ship. This splintering of responsibility for the daily work of the ports effectively prevented improvements in methods of working and equipment that a single employer would have made it his business to introduce. With the almost incredible working arrangements by which responsibility for ship turnround was often physically divided at the ship's rail between two employers, with workers belonging to separate unions and lightermen to a third, and with a powerful body of tally clerks intervening, how could there be a united surge towards better turnround? The aims and ambitions of all port employers are not directed to quicker ship discharge and loading. Where the profits of a private stevedore were made out of extra charges incurred or alleged, then undue haste would reduce the opportunities for these. With the drastic reduction in their number there is, today, a far healthier outlook between the few remaining stevedores whether port authorities or private firms. The pooling of expensive equipment and knowledgeable supervisory staff has been among the earliest of benefits.

Creeping Obsolescence of Premises

But in many ports progress has been crippled by long leases; modernization of areas, long overdue, is postponed until the premises can make way for new installations. An outstanding example of major dock areas which, elsewhere, would by their size constitute viable and independent ports and which have now outlived their usefulness and have ceased to exist, are the London and St. Katharine and the East India Docks in the Port of London. More will be said later on the important principle behind these closures. Many ports abroad are seriously handicapped because their industrial hinterland is not penetrated by an estuarial river, by tributary rivers, or canals on which a host of overside receivers can relieve the major harbour of the congestion that threatens every port that relies on working cargo entirely over its quays.

The introduction of the larger cargo unit will be looked at in some detail later. Port authorities who stand to benefit by exploiting this principle can attract cargo in larger sets by reduced handling rates; they can provide, at the door of the shed, a service of palletization for shippers of homogeneous cargo in the absence of palletization at an earlier stage.

A Static Industry

The first decade after the Second World War saw more changes, and the promise of major changes to come, than any preceding period in the history of the world's ports. Port construction from the beginning of the nineteenth century proceeded at a leisurely pace. The object was simply to produce more installations of a proved and accepted design but bigger and better than before. On this formula, berths that were provided in ever-growing numbers were occupied by the larger steam-vessels. By the early 1900s these had driven sail from all but the smaller ports. Improvements in quay cranes and ships' gear were made, electricity replaced hydraulic power and steam, but the fact remained that dock work was very much a static industry. The mid-Victorian introduction of the treadmill as the motive power for lifting cargo out of a ship's hold was hailed as a notable and very early step towards mechanization. Output per man and output per gang hour had only marginally improved between 1895 and 1945. The electric truck, brought into dock use in the early 1920s, was used in its same form 20 years later.

Post-war Outlook

Under the spur of wartime conditions, when mountains of warlike stores and ammunition had to be transferred from ship to shore without the intervention of a modern quay, the impossible was often achieved by the forklift truck, the mobile crane, the conveyor, and the tractor and trailer. To exploit these a new mentality made itself felt. Pre-war work had been attempted only under perfect conditions. The hand truck was master on the concrete quay. Generations of dockers had not conceived of conditions of work where this would not continue to be the reigning principle. The realization was quick to come that handling cargo units mechanically, instead of manually, had suddenly released the industry from the stranglehold of the manual labourer, a condition which, since Noah loaded his Ark, had been accepted. Within a few years the kinds of cargo that could be carried in bulk, and even in homogeneous units, were determined. All this progress was leading in the one direction—the introduction of the container, the eventual general cargo unit in weight and in size. To say that the container has introduced as many problems as it has solved is a truism that will be examined later. What is fundamentally true is the shattering release that the container has provided from the conventional and the traditional method of running the world's ports. The purpose and the function of a major container port, and the number of these that world traffic will be able to support, is not yet by any means established; the role may be reserved for a very few of the present major terminals. There is the general feeling, however, that no port can afford to ignore the spread of containerized cargo nor can it afford to be ignored when the general pattern of the international traffic takes shape.

Gradual Nature of Container Revolution

Whatever the doubts and the difficulties of port authorities and shipping companies over containers and whatever predictions are made and subsequently modified on the effect of container traffic on port labour and port usage, the fact remains that this is not a change that will come about overnight. The first post-war conversion of the wartime LSTs (landing ship, tanks) into commercial vehicle ferry ships was heralded in 1957 by the more enthusiastic as condemning the general cargo carrier to the horse-and-buggy age of transport.[1] That this did not happen is now general knowledge. Experienced port operators do not look for revolutionary change to take place because they know that no part of the port industry can ever be an island sufficient unto itself. Containers can be handled, it is true, as large boxes of general cargo. Within this limited field their effect on port work will never be of a nature to close down docks nor to make thousands of port workers redundant. This will only come about when special container ships have been constructed to carry the containerized imports by the many thousand tons, when special berths have been built and expensively equipped, and when this expensive process has been matched at the overseas ports. Where a shuttle service can be run within the same Customs enclave as between California and Hawaii, the operation is relatively simple and door-to-door transport has been achieved. When a liner loads cargo for a dozen ports and discharges, with intermittent coastal loading, at as many ports abroad, the turnover to container traffic is a far more complex and deliberate business.

Roll-on Ferry Ships

Whilst port authorities will continue to struggle with general cargo for many years to come, the roll-on ferry type of ship will become more popular (Fig. 2). The cost to the shipping company for cargo handling consists of a modicum of supervision only. The turnround time enables several voyages to be made during each day, and there is every attraction for containers to be carried as separate vehicle loads. When the time from a factory in the Midlands to a receiver in Milan can be measured in hours, how can conventional break-bulk shipping, with its delays in the dock shed at loading and in the transit shed at discharge, compete? No wonder that ports favourably placed such as Dover have increased their ferry traffic four and a half times in 12 years.[2] Similarly, bulk cargoes have made inroads into accepted handling methods. The integrated port where the raw material is discharged into a quay-side installation and processed there for export, probably to ships loading within the same port, has

[1] A Dutch port operator, after watching an early ferry operation, came away saying: "I have been looking at the stevedore's grave."
[2] In 1967 Dover shipped 191,000 tons in 34,663 units and received 361,000 tons in 20,171 units.

come to stay. Not only is the road, rail, and barge transport that was previously necessary to transport the raw material to an up-country manufactory not any longer brought into play, but capital is saved in the unnecessary payment of import duties, afterwards to be recovered on drawback. Documentation is simplified; loss by pilferage and damage disappears.

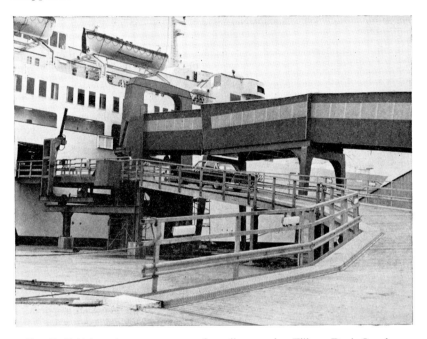

Fig. 2. Vehicle and passenger ramps for roll-on service, Tilbury Dock, London.
(By courtesy of PLA.)

Akin to the integrated port is the port where export processing zones are included. Here selected industries produce goods for export on ships berthed within a short distance of the factory. As well as the valuable tax and Customs privileges these industries enjoy, there are the obvious savings in transport and the costs of insurance. If we regard the ship as the transportation machine and the factory—in this case—as the job, we have here a good example of how advantageous it can be to take the job to the machine.

Approach to Port Problems

Accompanying this attempt at improving the turnround of general cargo ships there are a number of factors that are already making themselves felt. Several of them are valuable because they project a different mental approach to the problem. Compared with the equanimity and the complacency with which cargo-handling problems were tackled prior to 1939, this difference of approach—and it includes both sides of the industry—is as significant as any of the more obtrusive physical changes. The new type of port is now taking shape. Container berths, where the old facilities would guarantee the turnover of 100,000 tons per year, are now able to cope with one million tons per year although the area required is substantially greater. On the management side there is readiness to tackle problems from which their predecessors have shied for generations.[1] Decasualization, to the desirability of which every government inquiry into the running of British ports has subscribed since the Shaw Award of 1920, has now been introduced. Despite its teething troubles, no one would wish to put the clock back. Modernization is very much in the air. "You can, because you think you can" is now taking the place of that hoary, but immensely comforting, principle, "we have never done it that way before".

Labour's New Look

For generations the docker has protected himself against casual work and the evils of unemployment by restrictive practices. To spread the work he has refused to consider shift work. The difficulties of this are very real, and the greatest of them has always been a refusal to consider how the practical objections could be overcome. To disrupt the daily work by frequent stoppages or to manufacture disputes over piecework interpretations did little harm to the worker. The work was there when he was ready and willing to take off his coat once more. In the immediate post-war years an entire ship could be paralysed because each of six gangs was one man short and the "milking" of one gang to make up the remaining five was not tolerated by labour. The work remained there—it could not run away—until the six gangs could be completed at the next call. When labour was scarce, the hoarding of gangs against the expected arrival of

---

[1] A major port authority has (October 1969) made the job of labour relations the sole occupation of one of its principal officers.

ships was winked at, although other ships might be short of gangs on this account.

In 1969 there are signs that both sides are taking a new look. Modernization programmes include the serious attempt to bring in a system of two shifts without the attendant cumbersomeness of a complex overtime payment. Agreement has been reached on working such overtime as may be necessary, and how this can be allocated on a fair rota and not on the "blue-eyed boy" basis. In certain areas of the port where conditions are favourable, the gang system, in its restrictive application, has been all but done away with. Piecework, which was one of the objects for which the dockers of 1889 fought the Great Strike and for the exploitation of which both sides have been struggling ever since, is now seen to have had its day. The modern container berth cannot be controlled by the rigid application of a piecework schedule designed for conditions and a mentality that is, happily, on the way out. To pay a good wage to a few specialists who are equipped to handle phenomenal tonnages and who are ready and willing to ignore the day of the week or the hour that the ship berths, is now seen to be essential to a traffic that represents the heaviest capital investment that the port and shipping world has ever known. At long last the lesson has been learnt that good cargo handling will eventually drive out bad, and that the loss of traffic where old conditions are allowed to remain may be quicker than many of the diehards believe. A few years ago nothing could have seemed more permanent than the pattern of port working. An alternative to the gang of dock workers, complete with cargo hooks, was unthinkable. The changes that port workers have themselves seen and at many of which they have assisted, have been reinforced by the progress made by many small ports, some of which in the past were merely Edwardian summer resorts. Most of this traffic has come from—or being new traffic, would have gone to—the older ports. It has bypassed these and has enjoyed a freedom from labour disputes and stoppages that have consistently eroded the business still coming to the major ports. Now the simple lesson has been learnt by the younger and more flexible dockers that traffic lost is hard to regain, that no one has done more to make the dock worker redundant than he has himself, and that the long-term aim of every responsible party in commerce is the reduction in the tonnage of gang-handled cargo. He can see in a modernized and revitalized industry a future for himself not only when the containers do take over but during the years of transition. There is a willingness everywhere to be trained for special duties and a readiness by employers to provide the training pro-grammes that will ultimately lead to a flexibility of labour hitherto un-known. It has long been a reproach that dockers do not come to the dock to work; they come to see that agreements are kept or, better still, how they can be exploited to their advantage. If conditions are not in accordance with national or local agreements, work will not begin. If the lighterman or the tally clerk is not present when work should commence, men will remain idle. If the gang is not complete it will not make a start. If the weather is not favourable, output will be interrupted. Because of this new approach the picture of dock workers, determined to overcome these and similar obstacles so that the work can go on, is nearer today than it has ever been.

Provision of Amenities

For generations the conditions in which the dock worker was expected to handle cargo, harsh and inhospitable as they inherently were, had no background of local amenities which would have made them tolerable. Within living memory dock latrines went no further than a pole suspended over an open sewer with head cover in the more modern types. Today the provision of amenities in ports has now reached a level comparable with those provided by factory management. Despite, or perhaps because of, its dangers and discomforts, dock work should be regarded as deserving the comfortable conditions of the factory in so far as these are practicable; this is being belatedly recognized.

Function of the Port Authority

On the management side there is increasing recognition that the part they have to play in making the port efficient is not one of sitting on the fence, however excellent a landlord they have been trained to be. The port authority today must take the lead. It must recognize that it has a part to play in the economy of the country. As well as a reasonable expenditure on research (the setting up of a working committee to detect and to tackle port customs that restrict output suggests itself as a worth-while measure) it is necessary that port management should take an interest in what other ports, and not only those of their own country, are doing. What are the policies that determine the running of the ports of foreign countries, what are their intentions by way of development, of training for staff and labour, and do they see their future in terms of general cargo, of containers or bulk traffic or of an integrated port? In the past port authorities tended to over-centralize. Initiative and a new outlook were frowned upon by a management that discouraged enterprise and demanded only strict adherence to the book of rules. It is true that very few substantial suggestions for improving the enterprise were ever received from the staff of these ports. Men were taught to keep their eyes down at all times, and it was not surprising that a worm's-eye view was all they perceived. Before they can produce ideas of value, staff must first be encouraged and trained, and this is not a quick process. It is first necessary to engender the destructive habit among executives of asking "Why?"

The Benefits to the Efficient Port

A port efficiently run brings ample reward. It attracts full ships, and this includes vessels with cargo for transhipment to other ports. The optional traffic of pre-war years made London the distributive centre for several of the continental countries with not only visible, but invisible, benefits to English commerce. Coastal shipping, lighterage, insurance, and other fringe industries did well out of the entrepôt traffic that major ports attracted. With some ingenuity, the Far Eastern port of Kaohsiung has broken new ground in the manufacture of plywood. Imports of round mahogany logs from the Philippine Islands are discharged there and, at minimum expense, rafted directly overside and then taken by water to the plywood factory. The finished product, in bales, is then taken by craft to the export vessel in which it will leave the port. At no time has the raw material or the finished article been outside the Customs fence—costs of transport could not have been less and the generally accepted commercial risks have been eliminated. By such means, and by breaking new ground of this kind, the port is flourishing.

As an extension of the new kind of policy one cannot ignore the inland port. This principle is applicable where natural conditions such as a mountainous hinterland prevent the natural extension of the port area inland. At considerable cost, all the cargoes of incoming vessels would be transferred by road and rail to a depot area some few miles from the port. Here they would be sorted and delivered and, probably, there would be provision for warehousing. Such ideas as these, and they are by no means impracticable, are a far cry from the conventional port with its fixed berths.

The shape that the efficient port will take must vary with local conditions and the demands of traffic. No doubt under systems of nationalization, of which more will be said later, attempts to determine these will be made on a national basis. The future of many ports will then become bleak, for there is no doubt that there are at present far too many ports, and that as the outline of container ports becomes more definite, more ports—not only in this country but all over the world—will become redundant. To a lesser degree every port will have to examine its purpose and its future from a fresh angle. In London the inescapable truth has had to be faced that modern conditions of shipping leave no place for the early Victorian type of dock. The only remedy is the surgical cure of amputating whole areas from the modernized port, and this has already been done. Most ports will discover they have parts that cannot be brought up to date but which can, with advantage, be sold for housing or industrial purposes. They were built to meet certain demands. Time has replaced these with other requirements which the older dock areas cannot meet. They will have to go.

Air Freight

A cloud no bigger than a man's hand, but which will grow larger as the years pass, is the inroads being made by air freight on goods previously carried by sea. More will be said of this later.

Additional Note

Chapter 1, page 4, footnote 1. Taken from a publication of the Port of London Authority on Tilbury Dock.

CHAPTER 2

THE BERTH

Introduction

The ship berth is the most important single construction in a modern port. On its capacity and on the efficiency with which it is operated depends the speed of ship turnround. *The output of the port is the sum of the outputs at its several berths.*

The port is the installation that enables water-borne cargo to be transferred to land carriage; the berth is the point at which this transfer takes place. It is therefore the vital link in the transportation chain that stretches from producer to consumer. The speed of loading or discharging vessels determines the berth occupation or utilization, commonly known as the throughput of the cargo. This speed is directly governed by the rate at which labour can make up sets of cargo from the quay for stowing in the ship, or break-down sets of cargo taken out of the ship, for delivery or removal from the quay. This rate is the result of several factors; the efficiency of the port follows directly from the success with which the problems that surround these factors have been solved.

Berth Requirements

The present berth has developed from the hard standing on which the native coracle of the remote past was made fast. The fundamental conditions which were found there are still essential to the highly developed vessels of today. The general cargo berth demands, firstly, a deep-water quay alongside which is a constant level of water or where tidal conditions do not inhibit the working of a ship. In an enclosed dock this is ensured by impounding; if the tidal range is small, that is the good fortune of the port authority who are thereby saved the heavy cost of locking and impounding. There must be enough bollards or other means of holding the ship in all weathers with the minimum surging. Secondly, covered premises or open spaces for the shore handling of cargo must be adjacent to the quay, and if it is the custom of the port to work cargo with quay cranes, the quay surface—which should preferably be smooth—should carry a portal crane track unless mobile cranes are used. The berth should include a transit shed and, in addition, a general cargo warehouse for the long-term storage of staple cargoes. This should be situated in relation to the quay so that cargo can be worked directly to and from the warehouse and the ship. If the berth is used by ships bringing goods that do not need to be protected from the weather, i.e. softwood timber or containers, the housing or transit space may consist of open ground. In course of time the general berth with its attendant transit shed has been developed to include the special installations to handle the cargo of ships carrying frozen meat, bananas, grain, or sugar in bulk, etc. It has become a specialized berth.

Thirdly, the facilities that surround the berth are important. A berth may become sterilized because it is so placed as to make it difficult for an incoming vessel to tie up alongside in safety because of the prevailing wind or tidal conditions. It may be cramped in that there is not enough space for the vessel to work satisfactorily on a dummy nor for small craft to work ahead or astern. The end berth on a long linear quay is often thus handicapped, particularly when there is a vessel working on the adjacent cross-quay. Similarly, there is need for room for both road and rail vehicles to work freely. With the development of the rail-connected berth of the mid-nineteenth century, it did not take long to discover that the work of the berth nearest to the marshalling yard was liable to be interrupted by shunts made to clear and to supply berths further down the lineal quay. Intermediate approach and take-off points from a running line is the only satisfactory solution to this problem. Road traffic to a berth that specializes in immediate delivery goods such as fresh fruit is at a disadvantage if it is too far from the main dock gates or if it is situated in between export berths that attract heavy road traffic.

Restrictions on Output

The history of dock construction shows a very clear trend in creating conditions that induce a better output at the individual berth. This has not followed the same pattern in all ports. What can be done to increase the tons handled per gang hour is governed by many major factors. In the few ports that consist entirely of roadsteads where 100 per cent of the cargo is discharged into or loaded from craft, improvement can be gainfully directed to the turnround of the craft that keep the cargo from or to the ship moving. The largest and the most varied operation of cargo handling from ships a few miles out at sea was undoubtedly the supplies side of the Allied combined operations of the Second World War. No practical officer was surprised to find that the ship off a hostile beach, for whose discharge he was responsible, was handicapped by the chronic shortage or irregularity of arrival of craft. Similarly, to serve a general cargo vessel with road vehicles so that at no time does a set of cargo await a lorry in which to put it, is an almost impossible task; likewise, to keep a ship's cargo moving, even in an enclosed dock, when the sole outlet consists of craft, is almost impossible unless there is a surplus of craft, tugs, and lightermen on a scale that would make the job uneconomic. The craft problem is all important in this type of port. Improved ships' gear that could double the tonnage to be lifted would not advantage the turnround.

The Land-served Port

It is not strange that the same strait-jacket constricts the vessels that are compelled to work all their cargo ashore. Most of the western European ports have been built on the estuaries of major rivers; many of them serve a complex of waterways that are vital to the industrial hinterlands. Few of the Mediterranean ports are built on the estuaries of navigable rivers; many of them are hemmed in to a narrow coastal shelf by high mountains which are not easily penetrated by rail or road systems. Very few ports enjoy the inestimable advantage of being served from hundreds of miles around by the triple and parallel arteries of river, road, and railway, as can be observed in the Rhine industrial area. To be faced with a single outlet from a port—that of land carriage only—means that the port authority must give urgent consideration to providing the necessary alternative of water transport; albeit, this is only for an internal port movement. No port can prosper nor develop if the whole of its cargo has to pass over the quays. Where there are to be found a combination of perfect weather conditions, where the nature of the cargo is satisfactory, where there is ample labour and at all times the assurance of sufficient road and rail transport and the certainty of getting it into and out of the port without hindrance, then and then only could the entire discharge of cargo ashore be attempted with some prospect of success. Every practical man is taught by experience to expect the worst in port work; he is rarely disappointed. He knows that the above conditions will never come together or, should they do so, it will not be a conjunction on which he can base the next day's work. Ports like Rijeka in Yugoslavia and Keelung in Taiwan come to mind where nature has not only deprived the port of an outlet by water but has made road and rail traffic very difficult. In these circumstances the only solution is to introduce an internal lighterage system, and this can best be done by the port authority.[1] For this a fleet of barges, a few tugs, and—most important of all—one or more road- and rail-served lighter berths, will be necessary together with the organization to control both the supply of barges and their turnround at the lighter quays. This will mean spending money to provide a service for the speedier turnround of ships in the port, but the port authority will probably be farseeing enough to subsidize this service in their long-term interests. There may, as is the case wherever the custom of the port is first broached, be opposition from shipping companies and from receivers or shippers on the grounds of the double handling that lighterage involves, but this should disappear as the benefits of quick delivery become apparent. The kinds of cargo passing through the port and which lend themselves to lighterage will soon become apparent once the internal lighterage is in the hands of the port authority. The single ownership of barges makes it possible to standardize types and capacity as well as providing tugs of economic build. There is every encouragement for receivers to reduce costs by setting up waterside premises wherever practicable.

Ways of Working Cargo

The quickest turnround of a break-bulk cargo ship is obtained by a judicious manipulation of the available means by which the cargo is put into or taken out of the ship. It would be exceptional to be able to employ more than two gangs in each hold for discharge when this is made completely overside. Similarly, a ship that worked two or more gangs per hold ashore would, even starting with an empty shed, soon come to a standstill. The balance that a well-equipped berth enables the port operator to strike between cargo that can be landed and that which can be put overside, is provided by his essential "know-how" that his job has taught him. No amount of paper-work nor the production of graphs or "tonnage per foot run of quay" (as beloved by the British War Office) is a substitute. His know-how will be built on his constructive understanding, firstly, of the kinds of cargo he will have to handle, and, secondly, on the proportion

[1] See Appendix I.

of shore to overside receivers. If there are not enough of the latter he will be well advised to "invent" some by using internal lighterage.

Physical Factors of a Berth

These are the general principles that govern the working of every berth. Half a century ago it was exceptional to find other than the conventional general cargo berth, however, many minor variations there were in the design of this. Today it is almost the exception for new berths to be built that do not cater for a special traffic. Experience has taught the builders of the older docks that some improvement could be made as each opportunity for new construction came along. A student of dock buildings can quite easily read the signature of the engineer who designed each particular building and can tell at a glance the stage in the search for the quicker turnround of ships that the particular quay, shed, or warehouse illustrated. About 1914 the idea was mooted that you could not have too many delivery cranes for upper floors of transit sheds. To prove this—it did just the opposite—a shed was built which had delivery cranes placed at intervals of a few yards all along the upper floor. Quite one-third of the working space was taken up by internal staircases and crane boxes. Not more than a quarter of the cranes at any one time were ever seen to be in use. To provide permanent dummies for the discharge of ships in the King George V Dock, London, designed prior to 1914 but not opened until 1921, seven pontoons, each imprisoning four quay cranes, were placed along the lineal quay on the south side of the dock. Whilst providing all-round working for each ship, each berth was enclosed in a rigid pattern of quay cranes that effectively prevented adding to their number when required by fleeting more cranes along the quay track. Examples could be multiplied from every port in the world. It is the most difficult of all constructional berth work to prevent a good idea from deteriorating into a "folly"—and few major ports can boast of not possessing several of these.

The building of each berth must of necessity be empiric. Commencing at the water's edge, how wide should you make your quay? Here, again, one can point to the quay a few yards wide covered by the several floors of the warehouse of which it is a part. It was built to prove that goods could be landed from the adjacent ship and taken directly into storage. It proved nothing of the kind because the prevalent need for sorting to marks on all incoming cargo was overlooked. Conversely, there are quays in the port of Manchester where the working space for receiving softwood extends as far as 100 yards from the water's edge. In the days when all cargo landed was hand-trucked, extra payment was made for trucking beyond an agreed distance, and this was a factor powerful enough to restrict the width of many quays. With the new container berths it is idle to talk in terms of quay width; rather is it a storage area where the number of acres required has still not been determined.

There has been an argument over the layout of rail lines ever since berths were (more than 100 years ago) equipped with these. Assuming that it has been proved, and this will not be easy, that the traffic of the port includes enough rail-borne cargo to be handled directly into or out of rail wagons to warrant the expense, it is still a fact that rail traffic is declining in most ports in favour of road. Because of this there is a growing tendency to banish the rails to the rear of newly constructed sheds. With the development of container berths there will be scope for the delivery of containers to the berth by rail, but the layout will be different from the three-line system beloved by many earlier port operators. Seeing that ports are generally built on marsh or unstable land, there is always a tendency for wide spaces such as are required for ample rail facilities to subside in part; repair is expensive.

There has been development also in the type of quay crane from the hydraulic that replaced the hand crane to the modern level luffing electric. The portal quay crane that spanned one or more rail lines is giving place to the tripod type that can be placed on quays where there are no rails. Apart from argument over types and loading capacities, there is now the major contention as to whether the fixed or semi-movable quay crane has not been out-dated by the mobile crane. The basic fact in using a crane to discharge or to load a ship is that it should be available at the time required and for the working hours that it is needed and also at the hold where it is wanted. The number of cranes on the quay before the need arose or after the need has been met, is irrelevant save that no port has ever solved the problem of having all the cranes that shipping companies require during the time they want them. Unsolved also is the question of how to find work for the many unwanted cranes when the port is semi-idle. It is a classic instance of taking the job, in this case the ship, to the machine—the crane-equipped berth. Where the problem of working a ship by suitable mobile cranes has been solved, then it is possible, at great saving to the port authority and to the satisfaction of the shipping company, to take the machine to the job. Unlike the semi-fixed quay crane, the mobile crane can be used elsewhere as soon as its work on a ship is finished. With a practical usage of 312 days in a year (less a few for periodic maintenance), the number on which a mobile crane is unemployed is, and will always be, lower than that for the present type of portal crane. A glance at the quays of any major port, where large capital assets stand unused for days on end, will demonstrate this point.

A minor facility that speeds ship turnround is a satisfactory supply of dummies. These can give a flexibility to the discharge, particularly where there are quay or mobile cranes with sufficiently long jibs.

The Quay Shed

The quay shed is no exception to the universal rule that every building, from St. Paul's Cathedral to a dug-out in the trenches of the First World War, is a means of enclosing space that is needed for a particular purpose. In this case the need is protection from the weather not only for the cargo but also for the workers, room for putting cargo down to marks and sizes, room to sort and possibly to sample, for inspection also by Customs officers; and, in the past, but heavily frowned on today, room to house minor offices for staff, oilers' boxes, wash-places for men, and space to keep the tackle and gear needed for working the cargo. These are some of the prime requirements that a dock transit shed should meet. The emphasis must always be on the transit function of the shed. Through lack of understanding and through fear of upsetting powerful interests, some port authorities have allowed transit sheds to be used for the temporary housing of cargo which changing market conditions make it attractive for the merchant to leave there on rent. This is the quickest way of bringing a port to a standstill—as many ports in the Middle East have discovered. Unless special cargo is being handled, such as meat or bananas, the plainer and the less obstructed a transit shed can be kept the better it will do the job for which it was built.

Over the years there have been improvements on the simple transit shed, originally having dimensions of 400 ft long and about 130 ft wide and with about 10 ft of practical working height. There has been argument over how many floors a modern shed should have. It has been substantially resolved in favour of a ground floor for import cargo, the first floor for exports with protruding or recessed verandahs (the former give protection from rain to men working below), and the second floor for long-term housing and probably bonded for dutiable cargo. Access to the first floor

for vehicles may be by external ramp and these may commence not necessarily alongside the shed (Fig. 3). The cost of getting cargo upstairs and
down again may have to be taken into account. Wall cranes are slow moving
and cargo-lifts take up working room inside the floors; time is lost when
they have to return empty for another load.

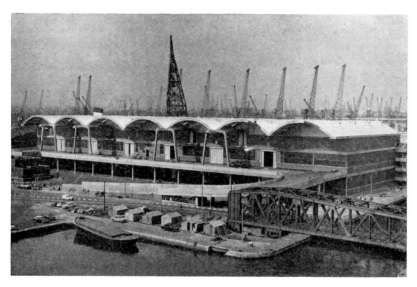

FIG. 3. M Shed, SW1 Dock, London; transit accommodation on ground-
and first-floor levels with ramp access for vehicles. Succeeding import vessels
discharge into alternate floors. (By courtesy of PLA.)

Modern cargo handling is founded on the pallet and the forklift truck,
with height being as important as area. Suitable cargo can be piled 20 ft
and more high by this means, and the tonnage accommodated can be
trebled as against manual piling.

Delivery banks were, until recently, considered an essential part of the
transit shed. For generations, rail wagons and lorries have been loaded
in this way, and it took some courage in the immediate post-war years
to accept the argument that the forklift truck had made the rail bank unnecessary. Where it had for so long been an asset it was now found to be
an obstruction. Reliance on rail delivery banks has now gone. The area

at the rear of the shed covered by rail lines should not be left "proud", but levelled over so as to give extra space for loading lorries.

To avoid extra trucking, sheds built right up to 1939 were provided with doors on to the quay at intervals of a few yards. Even before the arrival of the forklift truck, which abolished the bogey of distance, it was found that every door was made an excuse for a gangway and that this took up revenue-earning space whilst contributing nothing. The fewer there are the more cargo the shed will take. Suitable dimensions for doors are 30 ft wide by 20 ft high. Cargo can be piled on pallets and these can be reached either from the front or the rear of the stacks.

As sheds are quite often used alternatively for import and export cargoes (sometimes both are accepted into the shed at the same time), it is clear that any method of marking out floors must make provision for both.

If particular areas are reserved for export and import cargoes, then there is no problem of dual floor markings. If, however, the whole space is used at different times (or at the same time) for both imports and exports, then the export floor marking must be easily distinguishable from the import marking and vice versa. One method of doing this is by marking the corners only of export stacking areas; another is by using lines of a different thickness and/or of a different colour, or, again, by using broken lines. When a large proportion of exports is palletized, the export areas can be marked out in pallet sizes or multiples of pallet sizes, and these areas can be numbered as a means of locating cargo. Care must be taken, however, that floors are not over-marked, otherwise the attempt to avoid confusion will end by creating it. What *must* be clearly marked are the gangways. Obviously both the shed construction and the manner of its use have to be taken into account when deciding on gangways, but in the majority of cases only two or at the most three permanent gangways are really necessary, and, again, in the majority of cases 12–13 ft is the maximum width required although it is quite common to see gangways of between 13 ft and 18 ft. Additional gangways are, of course, desirable when circumstances permit, but they should be regarded as temporary amenities only to be given up when necessary. An actual shed plan is shown (Plan 1) to illustrate to what extent gangways can be allocated to get a maximum amount of stacking space.

In every port the demands of the national Customs have to be taken into account, and the situation may arise where parts of a multi-storeyed quay shed are bonded. It is advisable that floors should be bonded separately

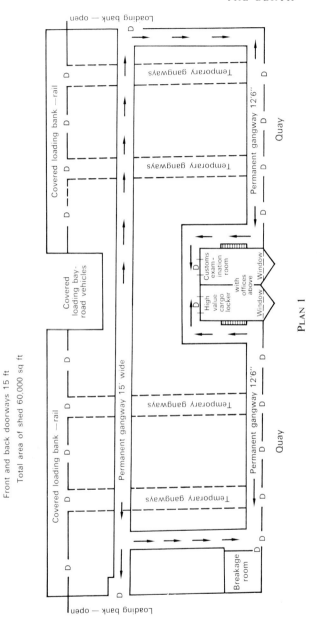

Shed layout

Size of shed 400 ft × 150 ft

D = Doorways. End doorways 18 ft

Front and back doorways 15 ft

Total area of shed 60,000 sq ft

PLAN 1

and not in parts, and that the whole shed should be owned by the port authority who are the body responsible for the integrity—from the Customs' view point—of the building.

The Warehouse

Warehouses have a part to play in ship discharge. Although their main function is to receive cargo for housing which may well be brought there by craft, it is quite practicable for homogeneous cargo in bags or cases, to be passed across the quay and lifted into the upper floors of warehouses situated, as is usual, in the rear of the transit sheds, and this at a rate that will keep the ship working at a normal speed (Fig. 4). Also in ports such as Amsterdam, Rotterdam, and Antwerp, where a manufacturing process goes on and much of the finished product is exported without leaving the port limits, the quayside warehouse fulfils the dual functions of transit and storage as well as processing.

Warehouses, where there is a rapid turnover of the cargo they house, have been built (in the Free Port of Copenhagen) with delivery loopholes that have been echeloned. This is an advantage over the vertical alignment because deliveries can be made with mobile cranes simultaneously from adjacent floors. Open sheds, equipped with overhead gantries, are normally provided for the handling of hardwood logs. This is a heavy capital cost and only partial utilization of the cranes is general. Mobile cranes, being transferable, will have a much higher use factor.

Work in the transit sheds, that are so essential as a part of dockland, is affected by the local rainfall. Some progress has been made since the Second World War in protecting berths. At the Swedish port of Skandia in 1967 a scheme was produced that provided ships to be berthed two at a time and on opposite sides of a series of bays so that the cover placed over each bay would protect two vessels at a time. This is a distinct advance on proposals for covering berths on lineal quays. Attention has, however, been very profitably concentrated on protecting the cargo, where this is homogeneous, rather than the ship. In the case of carcasses of meat for discharge, the elevators now used can be completely covered so that work can go on independently of weather. Similarly, in the rice-exporting countries of the Far East protection can be given by using enclosed helical chutes that handle bags delivered to them, by horizontal conveyor, from the warehouse store. Cement, a very vulnerable cargo, can be shipped during heavy rain in palletized units; each set is protected by an open-ended light plastic cover slipped over the top. This is removed as the pallet load is placed in stowage and then returned to the quay for further use. The work of receiving exports can be kept going during rain under the canopies that are now becoming standard equipment at either end of the modern export shed. Similarly, where barge berths form part of port activities it is not a difficult matter to protect the barges with a light canopy. The cost, and the value, of providing adequate weather protection, such

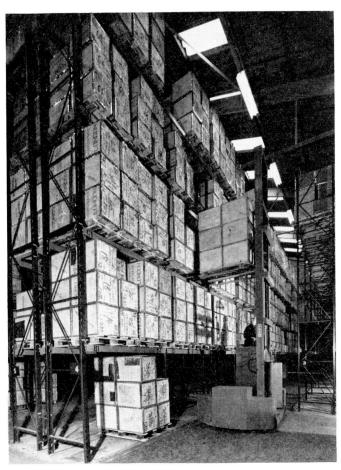

FIG. 4. Piling chests of tea in a modern fully automatic and computerized warehouse in London. (By courtesy of Buchanans Warehouses Ltd.)

as covered berths, will obviously vary considerably in ports situated in different parts of the world. A recent study was carried out by Arthur D. Little for the National Ports Council of the United Kingdom, and the method employed was published. Port authorities can now apply similar methods as an aid to reaching such conclusions as to the value of covered berths in their own ports.

General Points on Berth Usage

The arrival in 1946 of the roll-on ship as part of commercial shipping led to the construction of the very simple specialized berth that these ships require. It is merely an elaboration on the "hards" that were dug at right angles into the quay during the preparation in some United Kingdom ports for D-Day loadings, and on which the stern ramp could be lowered. It is disappointing to note that the owners of vessels employed on regular services have each specified installations that are particularly built to suit only their own vessels. There is no attempt so far to effect standardization of ramps or link-spans, so that the possibility of serving ports other than the usual ports of call is not likely to be easy.

Before leaving the physical aspects of the conventional ship berth there are a few points that need mention. Where there is a lineal quay, and this is still the accepted method of constructing ports, it is essential that there be a sufficient depth of water on each berth to allow a ship to work, or to move, whatever the state of the tide. It is often convenient to move ships during loading or discharge to make way for new arrivals. It has also been found that on a lineal quay of, say, six berths, the largest overall output will be obtained by a judicious mixing of import and export vessels. If, for instance, there are three export ships loading at a time, it would immensely congest the working of the quay if these were placed (reading from the main entrance) on berths numbers 4, 5, or 6. The closer they can be berthed to the sources used by the transport on which they depend for their cargoes, the better. On the other hand, if the cargoes of the import vessels call entirely for immediate delivery, as in the case of fresh fruit or bananas, precedence could then justifiably be given to these. A factor that counts is the number of rail wagons that each ship will attract and the consequent delays to road transport caused by frequent shunting. Obviously a ship with a cargo entirely for overside delivery would be given the berth at the further end of the quay. The bunching of ships and the unexpected delays in arrivals and sailings, so constant a feature of port work, will make the rational berthing of ships, as suggested above, difficult, and this has always to be accepted.

Some minor handicaps to good out-turn can often be seen in ports. There is always the problem of the heavy and awkward package which, it is hoped, can be delivered direct to rail or lorry. When this expedient fails, as it often does, the package has to be left on the quay; an accumulation of such obstacles can impede the free movement of gangs trucking cargo across the quay, just as crossing each other's path by import and export gangs working on the same vessel will do. This is often a sign of poor planning which has not made provision for the rational layout of the shed floor prior to the commencement of landing. In doing this all cargo known to be for immediate delivery should be bedded as near as possible to the delivery points, normally on the far side of the shed. The free flow of cargo is sometimes prevented by slow tallying, especially when this is caused by bad marking, making identification to bills of lading a slow and tedious job. There is surely a case here for the port authority to insist, through chambers of shipping and commerce, on a simplified marking system to be used by the shippers. The many marks borne by Cape oranges, shipped to Great Britain, and which slowed down discharge, have been appreciably reduced by a very simple code. Certain raw materials, such as cotton, hemp, and sizal, produced and shipped by individual growers, provide plenty of scope for introducing more easily identifiable marks. The very poor methods of marking bales of cotton has prevented the profitable use of forklift trucks from the ship's side. Where tallying has been a straightforward process, improvement in output has been obtained by abolishing the ship's side tally which causes an inevitable delay in the crane cycle, and replacing this by the "in-stack" system.[1] Here the tally is taken at leisure, either in the shed or on the piling ground.

It is not uncommon in watching work in a port to notice the poor state in which quays are maintained. Holes in the concrete and unevenness where the quay surface meets the inset rail, or gaps caused by the wear of truck wheels at door entrances, are a few of the signs that this aspect of berth out-turn has been neglected. In ports where there is much rain it is depressing for men to have to work through a series of puddles that have formed on low-lying parts of the quay. Unnecessary damage is caused to

---

[1] Port authorities and others who are interested in this system can obtain full particulars on application to the Central Office, ICHCA, Abford House, Wilton Road, London, SW1.

packages of fine cargo, such as occasionally fall off hand-trucks, in these conditions.

The revolutionary effect that mechanization of cargo handling has brought about on the berth will be dealt with later. It is sufficient here to stress that there should at all times be enough quay or mobile cranes, tractors, trailers, and forklift trucks and internal lighterage barges so that the equipment waits on the cargo rather than the reverse.

The Modern Specialist Berth

With the advances that have been made in recent years in the shipment of cargo in bulk, a new type of berth—foreign to conventional ideas—has come to be recognized. Apart from the abandonment of the accepted type of transit shed with its many doors and gangways, low roof, its clutter of offices and internal buildings, and its unnecessary delivery banks, provision has now been made to handle bulk sugar which, the world over, has almost entirely replaced shipment in bags by berthing the ship on a built-out jetty. From here, taken out of the holds by grab cranes, the sugar is transported by conveyor to the bulk storage ashore. As craft can be laid along the inner side of the jetty, the grab cranes can also work from or into these. Discharge of about 800 tons per hour is possible.

Since the first shipment of frozen and chilled meat into United Kingdom ports towards the end of the last century, it has been handled very much as general cargo. Discharge has been improved by using electric trucks and overhead runways, but weather and the human element have been twin deterrents to high output. The modern meat discharge berth is totally enclosed. The cargoes are taken out by elevators, handled henceforward on conveyors into an automatic tallying and sorting house on their way to the loading conveyor, and, finally, into the delivery vehicle. Aided by computers, each elevator (one per hold) can handle 100 tons of meat an hour.

The berth for bulk grain has not materially altered since bucket elevators replaced the primitive method of filling bags from the bulk by using wooden shovels. Recent improvements have vastly pushed up the output. These have included practical steps to keep up the discharge rate during the final stages in each hold, when output from the main plant falls off. It is, however, worth remarking on a custom of some ports that has limited the size of craft to 250 tons capacity. A barge of this size can be loaded in 15 minutes. The time of the valuable machines that serve the ship will be wasted whilst an empty barge to replace the full one is placed under the spouts. In many ports where barges carry up to 3000 tons, discharge is continuous.

The revolution in the import of timber that now arrives packaged instead of loose will be mentioned later. Here it is sufficient to say that the simplest form of berth—plenty of open space over which forklift trucks can manoeuvre is all that is needed. An outstanding example is the new timber

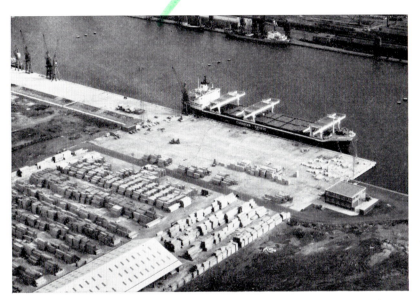

FIG. 5. Aerial view of mechanical-handling timber berth at Newport Docks. (By courtesy of British Transport Docks Board.) (The old system of handling timber is illustrated in Fig. 15.)

berth at Newport, which is 1400 ft long and 635 ft wide (Fig. 5). One shed, 736 ft long and 120 ft wide, provides under-cover storage for high-class timber. To allow for night work there are floodlight towers along the centre line, and, to iron out delays, each truck has two-way radio. An output of some 1300 standards, about 4000 tons, a day is possible.

Under-use of Berths

Despite the specialized berths with their high output, it is a fact that the majority of general cargo berths in the world's ports are not being used much beyond 30 per cent of their capacity. Firstly, few are worked for more than a single shift although this is often supplemented by a few hours' overtime. Whether this, if regularly worked, does produce more throughput than a normal 8-hour shift is a very moot point. There are practical reasons against working a three-shift day; the ancillary interests that serve the port are too powerful and too complex for a change to continuous ship loading or discharge to be brought in overnight. Secondly, rarely are quay cranes or ships' derricks used to the capacity of their full safe working loads. Three or five tons is demanded for the occasional lift, and this lifting power is now available for every lift. Unfortunately, sets of this weight of general cargo could seldom be made up in the ship's hold nor handled safely or economically on the quay. Over the years a mean size and weight for the general cargo set has been evolved. This works well, but it has condemned the crane cycle to but partial use of its capacity. It is, however, true that the larger cargo unit is breaking through the conventional straitjacket. On the modern container berth, work is continuous and each set—either a single container or two containers held

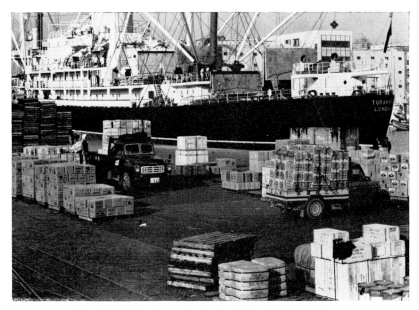

FIG. 6. Unit-load cargo being handled at Kobe Harbour.
(By courtesy of Japanese Information Centre.)

together—may quite likely reach the lifting capacity of the crane. There is still a long way to go before general cargo is handled for more than a moiety of its international volume, either in unit load form or by containers (Fig. 6).

It will be obvious that ports are now getting away from both the conventional berth design and the method of working that formed part of sailing-ship technique. Much of it has been founded on port customs, the most difficult of all working practices to breach; we have already spoken of these. Perhaps the port worker, and this includes executive as well as labour, has a deep and abiding love for the established practice by which his working life is ruled. He may not be aware of this: it is true, as pointed out in the report that followed one of the many post-war inquiries set up by the British Government, that the docker hates and will resist change even when it is to his advantage. This is probably true of other world ports. The improvements that can be noted since 1945 in the design and working of general cargo berths are still of an order that should raise a fundamental question in the minds of port operators everywhere.

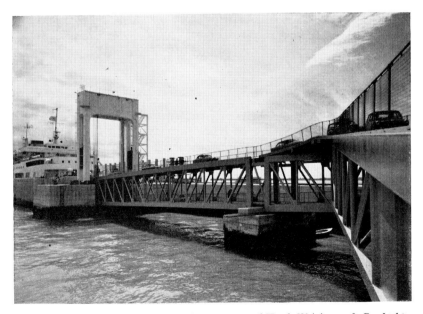

FIG. 7. Dover ferry with car ramp. (By courtesy of Head, Wrightson & Co. Ltd.)

The Need for New Berths

Is it worth building more berths until we have contrived to get a higher output from the existing ones?[1] To develop part of the port and to duplicate the present pattern, albeit incorporating a few modern improvements in the design, is an expensive job. There is, however, a great deal of interest and not a little glamour in the achievement (Fig. 7). To tackle the often dreary and always contentious job of improving output from present berths, has no glamour and very little attraction to management. If the existing berths that now give 30 per cent of their capacity could be made to produce 60 per cent—and this should not be impossible—then there would be no call to spend more money merely to perpetuate present inefficient working. A berth on which the management are content to work four gangs at the none-too-sparkling output of 20 tons per gang hour will have a throughput of only 640 tons in an 8-hour working day. By employing an internal lighterage system, where this is practical, at least two more gangs could be used to add to the output. By mechanization or other methods, the hourly gang tonnage could be raised to 30 tons, giving 1440 tons in the same working period. In other words one efficient berth is now doing more work than two inefficient ones did, with also—be it noted—a marked drop in overhead costs per ton handled.

---

[1] A new light has been shone on this problem by the successful discharge (July 1970) of LASH ships. A port, faced with new business handled in ships too large and deep for the existing facilities, can now berth the LASH parent ship in deep water outside the port limits; the cargo can be brought into the port in the LASH craft which can be discharged/loaded alongside the quays at no extra constructional expense to the port authority. It is now possible to *expand* the throughput of a port without *extending* the port.

Additional Note
Chapter 2, page 30, par. 4, Frozen meat. The first frozen-meat ship to reach England berthed at No. 4 Shed, East India Dock, in 1882.

CHAPTER 3

THE SHIP

THE previous chapter has shown how the berth—the natural home of the cargo ship—has developed from the primitive wharf to the specialized container berth. Parallel with this movement has been the process by which the conventional "three-castle" ship of the inter-war years has been outmoded by changes aimed at a quicker turnround in port.

Bulk versus General-cargo Ships

No man can see the final tonnage to which the bulk carrier will be built. Ships of more than 300,000 d.w.t. are already in service; shipbuilders are optimistic that this figure can easily be exceeded. Of the many difficulties of navigation and manœuvre predicted for super-sized vessels, none has so far proved insuperable. The aspect of ship turnround that makes such expansion profitable is the ease with which cargo can be loaded and discharged. Compared with general cargo there are, in fact, no problems. The contents of a bulk carrier are homogeneous, the complete shipload forms one bill of lading (hence there is no tallying nor sorting to marks and ports), labour for handling the cargo is not a problem, neither is the weather.[1]

Work can be continuous, supervision is nominal, and neither loading nor discharge is complicated by receiving or delivery from or to more than one source. Compare the time taken in shipping 10,000 tons of oil—a very small part of the cargo of a bulk carrier—with the complex process of loading the same tonnage of general cargo. It would be wearisome to catalogue the many stages through which the hundreds of separate bills of lading that would make up this traffic would have to pass; nor to mention the scurrying crowd of supervisory staff, labour, shipping agents, lightermen, tally clerks, and the like, who have to process the 1000-odd pieces of paper that have a part to play before the ship can sail.

[1] Although for some of the giant tankers experience has already shown that rough weather can prevent the tugs needed for berthing the ship from putting to sea.

Apart from the administrative side of the working of a conventional cargo ship, the size of the vessel that brings traffic to a berth, or takes traffic that has passed over the dock berth, has been determined partly by the shore facilities.[1] With running costs in port around about £1000 per day, it is not economic to attempt to load a ship with an excessive amount of general cargo. Both loading and discharge are still, in the main, slow and tedious jobs. The bills of lading taken into the ship on the first day would be very much delayed in arrival at their destination the longer the loading and discharge took. Again, probably half the cargo that goes into an export ship has, physically, to pass through the export shed. A substantial portion should be available to the loading stevedore before he begins his first day's work. Barges bringing cargo for the vessel have to be accommodated in the dock waters where berthing space is restricted. An import ship breaking bulk counts on having an empty transit shed; the major problem during discharge is to keep the cargo in the shed fluid by whatever means the port operator can devise. A shed that has been allowed to become congested will restrict the turnround of the ship by limiting the number of gangs whose output can be absorbed across the quay.

The major deterrent to larger cargo vessels is, therefore, the small unit of cargo; as this gives way to larger units and, eventually, to containers, there will be scope for increasing the size of the ships that carry them. Even so, a reasonable limit of 25,000 d.w.t. is envisaged as the extent to which it would be economic to assemble or disperse a cargo composed entirely of containers.

The depth of water in many ports and the impossibility often of dredging to greater depths will always restrict the size of the ships using them. Bulk cargoes can be piped or carried by conveyors to or from a jetty built out in deep water.

Changes in the Conventional Ship

A feature of the pre-1939 ship, to which little attention was paid by port operators, were the doors through which stores and victuals could be passed as required. After the Second World War a new and important use was seen as efforts were made to find new ways by which cargo could be taken into and out of ships' holds. The side port idea was developed, one of the first uses involving a mechanical transporter that could be run out

[1] An examination of the factors that determine the size of a vessel of the mixed cargo carrying kind is made in Chapter 10.

to plumb the quay and to pick up vehicles. Later moves have been in the direction of using forklift trucks to operate within the hold and to pass a unitized load through the sidedoor to a waiting forklift truck on the quay.[1] As it is able to receive cargo at varying heights, the forklift truck can marry up with its fellow in the hold as the ship rises or falls in the water.[2]

A variant on the side port was the access ramp by which vehicles could reach the interior of the ship from the quay. In the latest type of combined container and roll-on ship, vehicles enter through the stern doors. There is access to the two upper and two lower decks by internal ramps, along which the vehicles can be driven.

Changes in Cargo-handling Equipment, etc., on Board

Whilst retaining the conventional design, much thought has been given to including in this improved equipment that can be used to hasten turn-round. Lower decks have been strengthened to allow loaded forklift trucks to operate over them, and these are now carried by some ships as much a part of their handling gear as are the conventional winches. Standard construction now provides for flush hatches both on the main and the 'tween decks to give free play to these trucks.

As the value of the space directly under plumb came to be recognized and the loss represented by horizontal movement of cargo within the ship appreciated, the amount of space immediately below the hatches was sensibly increased by making hatches that were large enough to form an open-deck ship. A variant of this idea, and one which gave the shipworker more control of the space exposed to weather, was the double or triple set of hatches in line across the ship's beam and built over certain holds only.

To exploit the advantages of an open ship, the travelling gantry system was devised. This consists of a series of rolling-bridge cranes travelling on runway beams arranged along the length of both sides of the ship. Each rolling-bridge carries an extensible boom which can be extended to plumb beyond the ship's rails on either side of the vessel. The advantages claimed for this equipment are that every point within the open area of

---

[1] Some scope has been found for working cargo direct from rail wagons on the quay on to forklift trucks and thence through the ship's side door.

[2] The importance of the unit-load ship in ocean transportation is shown by plans to build six side-loading ships of between 15,000 and 20,000 d.w.t. for a regular unit-load service between Britain and Pacific Coast ports (April 1969).

the ship can be reached in the minimum time, the crane cycle is short, (as many as 60 per hour is claimed) and the outboard movement of cargo is done in the most efficient manner.

As parts of engineering installations overseas become bigger and heavier, the need has been felt for ships specially equipped with heavy lifting derricks that could both handle and transport these. A typical ship so equipped can make a lift of 300 tons from the quay. To prevent the vessel listing beyond the safe 12 degrees, there is an arrangement of tanks which can be filled with 3000 tons of fuel oil that can be used by the ship's engines, or with water. Part of the ballasting system consists of tanks for carrying vegetable oil or liquid tallow as cargo.

A major problem for shipowners has always been that of having to carry their own gear for use in ports which do not provide unloading or loading equipment to suit a specialized traffic. Many ports that welcome heavy lifts, such as containers, do not handle sufficient of these to make it worth while to provide the expensive quay cranes that are a feature of the modern container port. The ship gantry crane, usually mounted on rails set astride the hatch covers, has the advantage that high-speed loading or discharge can be done by the ship, thereby achieving an independence of whatever shore facilities are to be found in the port. Other advantages are that movement as between the ship and the shore crane is eliminated and with a shorter travel distance for the load. Container sway is reduced.[1]

As the pattern of world container traffic becomes clearer and the number of ports that are prepared to provide the expensive quay cranes increases, the gantry-equipment will tend to be used only on ships sailing at ports where shore-based equipment cannot be justified.

Not only are overseas engineering installations calling for means of transporting heavy loads by sea: in Great Britain certain units, notably transformers, for delivery to new power station sites, were proving impossible to carry by road; rail carriage was impractible owing to the outsize dimensions of many of these. The sensible solution was the transport of loads, some as heavy as 300 tons, by roll-on roll-off vessels specially designed for a traffic that would be sufficient to make their use economical. Since Manchester was the port nearest to some of the production centres, it was selected for this new business, although the building of a "hard"

[1] The utilization of ship-borne gear is, however, very low, and as the time spent in port by vessels is reduced by greater efficiency, so the hours when such gear can be used will also be reduced.

is all that is essential, and this can be done wherever there is suitable road access to a depth of 15 ft of navigable water. As most collecting points are near the coastline, the delivery of these huge units has been simple. The ships specially built are capable of carrying three unit loads at a time, together with one road transporter. The vessel's trim during loading and unloading is controlled by automatically operated ballast tanks. Parts of the load that are unsuitable for hold stowage, such as boiler drums, can be carried on deck. The *Aberthaw Fisher*, the prototype vessel on this service has now been joined by the *Kingsnorth Fisher* in the transport by sea of heavy indivisible loads over 90 tons.

Changes away from the Conventional Ship

In an article on mechanization that appeared in a technical journal in the immediate post-war years, the question was asked "Shall we ever get away from the tyranny of the cargo hook and the hole in the deck through which it works?" The building of larger ships that followed immediately after the Second World War seemed merely to accentuate the problem. The time taken to lift a set of export cargo from the quay and to lower it on to the ceiling of some of the newer ships was so long that the full gang, trucking out cargo from the shed, could no longer be fully employed. The crane cycle ceased to be an economic operation. The process was everywhere seen to be outdated.

The Roll-on Ferry Ship

Most of the simple ideas that have revolutionized cargo handling have not been exploited until they had passed their first youth. The container, the forklift truck, and the mobile crane were all in use in the inter-war years. The ferry that carried rail wagons from Reggio in southern Italy to Messina in Sicily was familiar to the grandparents of today's port operators. The landing ship, tank (LST), an adaptation of the simple ferry, played a real part in the amphibious operations of the Second World War, particularly in the Pacific area. Many port executives doing their job in khaki and watching the rate of turnround of these ships,[1] speculated on their peacetime uses. By 1947 a service of wartime LSTs started to run commercially from London with vehicles for the BAOR. Today there are

---

[1] In September 1943, with an average of 300 army personnel and a full load of tanks and armoured vehicles, an LST on the beaches at Salerno decanted this load within 20 minutes of lowering her ramp. This was a typical discharge under wartime conditions.

more than twenty regular services from ports in Great Britain to near-continental destinations. Apart from their appeal to private motorists, the modern ferry attracts cargo in the form of unit loads and containers on trailers (Fig. 8). Outsize loads are carried from door to door on lowloaders. The high-capacity forklift truck is used for loading and also for discharging large unit loads for transfer to continental lorries. Both heated and refrigerated units can be assured of electric points on board which will maintain

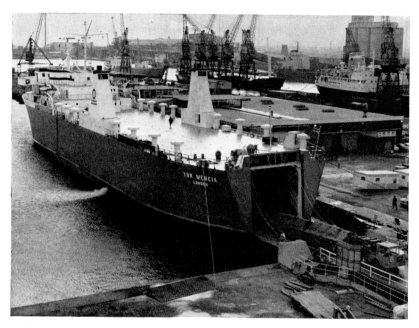

FIG. 8. *Tor Mercia*, Tor Line, on arrival at Immingham; first vehicles leaving.

temperatures at required levels. To make use of a strengthened upper deck, some modern ferry ships have had installed a 30-ton capacity hydraulic lift with a watertight hatch cover. On this type of ship general cargo can also be loaded by quay crane into the 'tween decks, through hatches fitted with single-pull covers.

The modern passenger/commercial ferry ship has accommodation for some 400 passengers, 100 cars belonging to these, 100 containers, and 500 tons of unitized cargo which is dealt with on large, flat trays moved by forklift trucks. This complete cargo, for which several days were previously required for the loading, can now be dispatched within one day. Before the speed and simplicity of loading and discharge of ferry ships had been appreciated, and this is particularly true of voyages that can be reckoned in hours, much play was made with the cubic space lost between the lorry or trailer floorboards and the deck of the ship. To a generation reared in the stowage of bags and small cartons where much labour and time can make certain of the minimum lost cubic space, the yawning gap inevitable with cargo on wheels seemed a retrograde step. However, doubts were soon dispelled when the economic picture of the modern ferry ship came to be examined.

The Articulated Ship

Based on the sound conception of the "iron horse" towing unit, proposals have been made for a cargo vessel that would include one propulsive unit to operate in conjunction with three (or more) cargo units. As a general-cargo vessel spends some 50 per cent of its working life in port it is obvious that the after-end of the vessel containing the engines, the bridge, and the crew's quarters waits on the convenience of the forward end containing the cargo, before it can resume its proper duties. This is a waste of capital and labour that has hitherto been accepted as inherent in ship construction. Varying with the length of the voyage, it is estimated that one cargo unit would be at either end of the conventional route and one unit in transit, attached to the propulsive unit. The work of three normal vessels would, it is claimed, be done at a cost of one-and-two-thirds that of a single conventional vessel. The subsidiary duty of operating a car ferry during the holiday season is also suggested for the power unit.

The LASH System

Whilst the container and the palletized load was receiving attention, the barge—as a vital link in ship turnround—was not neglected. A fully laden barge represents a cargo unit that is mobile and in which the cargo can be kept intact for long periods and can be protected from weather. As this desirable unit has hitherto only been achieved by the breaking down of the cargo in the ship's hold and its re-assembly within the hold of the barge, it was an obvious step to visualize a barge already loaded and placed within carrying space of a general-cargo ship. It was equally obvious that the conventional barge would not be suitable for hoisting into the conventional ship. It was true that lighters for transporting troops taking part in amphibious landings had been carried on ships' decks and lowered into the sea off hostile beaches, but their weight was not comparable with that of a loaded barge. A vessel of a new design, to be named LASH ship (lighters aboard ships), (Fig. 9) was produced, and 233 identical lighters are in production. Unlike the conventionally designed barge which has not altered since it was manually propelled by a lighterman with "sweeps",

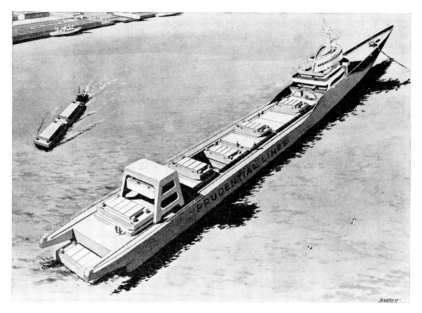

Fig. 9. Artist's impression of LASH ship.

the LASH barge is a rectangular box, $61\frac{1}{2}$ ft long, 31 ft 2 in wide, and 13 ft deep; it has a deadweight carrying capacity of 370 tons. Unitized cargo can be discharged from these by forklift trucks, and the LASH barges are ideal for containers. The "mother" ship can carry seventy-three barges on each voyage, and the full barges are discharged over a stern platform by the ship's own diesel gantry crane. As they are designed for working over inland waterways, they should shortly become a familiar sight on the European complex of navigable rivers and canals. Although conditions for discharge are more favourable in a harbour, it is claimed

that the system works equally well on a seaway.[1] A point of some importance is the saving in working costs that is anticipated. As the loading of
barges is a vital part of the turnround machinery of a general-cargo
ship, they are often worked during overtime hours so as not to delay the
ship. By getting rid of a cargo unit of some 350 tons in a matter of 25
minutes it is envisaged that the ship would turn round in hours instead of
days, and that the LASH barges could be discharged by their receivers
at leisure and without overtime costs.

There are certain developments promised from the original idea of
ships that carry barges. Space for heavy lifts, containers, and bulk cargo
has been planned, and there will be a total carrying capacity of some
27,000 tons. In so far as ships can arrange for the cargo they carry to be
unitized, the restriction on the size of general-cargo ships can be relaxed.
A limit of some 12,000 tons visualizes a ship in which cargo has to be
handled package by package. If by pre-shipment planning the "package"
can consist of a fully loaded barge, then the remarks made earlier on
time spent on loading and discharge will not be applicable. It could be
said that a ship of this kind is already knocking at the door of the
bulk-carrier trade.[2]

Ships for Special Cargo

A very natural development following from changes in the size and nature
of the unit of cargo has been the production of a ship suitable for the new
exports. In 1949 the *Baron Haig*, a ship whose name should go down in
history, carried 5000 tons of raw sugar in bulk instead of in bags. She was
an ordinary dry-cargo freighter, and for several years the sugar trade
attempted the impracticable—the economic loading of a bulk substance
into the holds of vessels designed—and not too cleverly at that—for odd-
shaped pieces of mixed cargo. The holds in all but the specialized ships of
the period consisted of irregular spaces of no known geometric shape,
combined with one or more shelves, known as 'tween decks, in which
cargo such as motor-cars or casks of wine could be given more attention
than they would get down below. The whole of the cargo space had to

[1] The 43,000 d.w.t. *Acadia Forest*, the first LASH ship, arrived in the Thames in
November 1969 with paper products from Mississipi mills.
[2] A design has been prepared (June 1969) for a "barge on board" (BOB) ship, the
main feature of which is that container barges enter a wet dock in the side of the ship
instead of over the stern. The containers are then hoisted into the holds by a travelling
gantry of 300-ton capacity.

conform to the shape of the ship, and this was built primarily to meet the needs of navigation and stability. It is small wonder that after struggling unsuccessfully to make the general-cargo ship a suitable carrier for bulk sugar which, during the voyage, turned itself into a solid and non-pulverulent mass, the sensible step was taken of building special sugar carriers. In these the grab, the method ultimately and only after many experiments, found to be successful, can work with the maximum freedom, and realistic tonnages can be discharged.

A few years after the *Baron Haig* had delivered the first bulk-sugar cargo in London, a smaller vessel sailed almost unnoticed into the Thames estuary port of Rochester. She carried a "bulk" cargo of softwood timber, the bulk being composed not of a hard mass of congealed sugar but eminently handlable packages of timber in deals and boards. Of this revolution in cargo handling more will be said later. Here it is enough to say that there are now specially built ships with a capacity around 17,000 d.w.t. that carry full cargoes of Columbian pine and can be discharged at the rate of 3000–4000 tons per day. This is possible because these ships are built with one continuous deck and six twin-hatched cargo holds arranged specially for carrying packages, each weighing around one ton. It is very doubtful if 16,000 tons of timber in loose condition would ever be shipped in that form. No experienced shipping company would face the delay both at loading and discharge of a possible 16 million pieces of timber each of which would have to be handled several times. Newsprint has always been a vulnerable cargo, both by damage in handling and by weather. Ships specially built for this traffic have deck gantries that span the holds. They are provided with clamps that not only pick up a complete load of rolls of paper but also give shelter, whilst in transit, against rain or snow.

Although not strictly speaking a ship, the "dracone", which is a flexible and towable container made from synthetic rubber-coated nylon fabric, can carry a load of liquid cargo in conditions that would be unsuitable for a decked vessel, and at a tithe of the cost of a propelled and crewed ship. The hovercraft, again on the borderline of the accepted ship design, has already made an impression on the motor-car carrying trade. It would indeed be ironic, but indicative of the speed of change in the industry, to see the post-war car ferry outdated by a more speedy carrier.

In March 1969 discussions were taking place in the United Kingdom with the purpose of increasing the size of hovercraft so that they could be used to carry export cargo. If their advantages of speed and flexibility could be exploited, it would mean a major breakthrough in the transport industry.

Nuclear-powered Ships

Although not directly related to its cargo-carrying capacity (and there has not so far been anything surprising in the method of handling this), the ship driven by nuclear power has come to stay. Since the American *Savannah*, the prototype vessel of this kind made her maiden voyage in 1962, progress has been slow. Early in 1968 a German-built nuclear-powered vessel came into full operation, making, with the Russian ice-breaker *Lenin*, the third ship of this kind. There are plans from the United States, Japan, and even China for further ships that will be nuclear powered. It is claimed that a container ship could so operate more economically than ships conventionally driven. In March 1969 the British Government instituted a preliminary survey into the economics of nuclear-propelled cargo carriers. There is little doubt that this will be followed by intensive research into the potential size of the market, the consequences of neglecting this development, and of what importance it would be nationally were it to be government supported.[1]

The Container Ship

The first stage in the thinking on carrying containers as ships' cargoes was completed when it was decided to divorce the new traffic from the category of "heavy lifts". This had, over many generations of port operators, become synonymous with the slow and deliberate handling of large packages by the heavy-lifting floating cranes maintained by port authorities as a necessary but uneconomic facility. Only in its weight did the container conform to the traditional heavy lift. To reap full advantage of the largest unit of general cargo that had been produced, it was necessary that speed of handling should be allied to the homogeneous nature of the new traffic. The standardization of dimensions made possible by the work of the International Standards Organization produced the cellular container ship where phenomenal outputs and intakes have become normal.

The traditionalists, having lost the first round, and having retired floating derricks into the obscurity from which they are only too seldom

[1] In October 1969 details of new designs for a nuclear-powered container ship of 43,000 d.w.t. to carry 1800 containers at a speed of 24 knots were being considered.

summoned, then endeavoured to arrange an unholy marriage between the general cargo and the container. A design for ships was suggested that would have allotted a proportion of the cubic space to containers and the balance to conventional cargo. One lesson that the most tradition-bound port operator had early learnt told him that the time taken to discharge a ship is determined by the rate of working of the slowest hold—a few hundred tons of awkward cargo stowed in the mid-ship's tanks can prevent a ship from keeping her sailing time unless the slow rate of discharge has been anticipated. Hence the fact that the combined container and general-cargo ship would never leave the berth until the last ton of mixed cargo had been taken out by conventional means, early became apparent.

An exception to this argument is the ship that has always carried a full general cargo and is equipped to handle this. One shipping line is now lengthening their vessels so that ninety containers, each 20 ft long, can be carried. These will be shipped and discharged more as large packages that are part of the general cargo, and will be out and away long before the massive tonnage of general cargo has been disposed of. This is an example of the difficulty of laying down the law in any port matter—there is always the exception. In this instance, as no attempt is made to integrate the handling of the containers and the main cargo, no contrary principle has been introduced.

A marriage that gives every sign of stability is the combined container and vehicle ship. The container, which is fast-moving cargo, is closely rivalled by the car or lorry driven in through the stern door.

The Unit-load Ship

The importance of the concept of the unit load is that it is a mass-production system applied to cargo handling. The flexibility of the pallet will always be advanced against the rigidity of the container, and it is not surprising that advocates of the former find much support in the unitized ships that abound in the Australian trade. Typical of these is the open-deck ship with twin- or triple-deck hatches abreast and equipped with electric cranes that can lift any load from a single pallet upwards; in some cases a 20-ton lift (Fig. 10).

The Bulk-cargo Ship

The reaction of the port operator of a generation ago to the modern bulk-carrier ship would have been one of sheer incredulity that it was

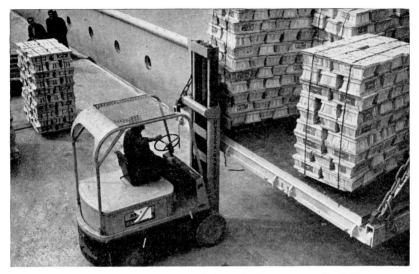

Fig. 10. Discharging fruit in unit loads through side ports on a Fred Olsen
vessel, Millwall Dock, London. (By courtesy of PLA.)

practicable and reasonable to build and navigate ships of a size that his
imagination had never entertained. However, there seems little hindrance
to developments that will produce the half-a-million-ton ship that would
have been outside the range of Jules Verne's conjecture. On one point
there is complete agreement—the bulk ship, save for the small types acting
as feeders for integrated industries working within a port area, will not
be able to enter an enclosed dock, nor, on account of their draught, can
they be accommodated within the ordinary port.[1] Exceptions are natural
ports such as Milford Haven where the main channel can be dredged to
give 65 ft of water and where nature has provided ample turning space.
Where it is advantageous for a mammoth tanker to be able to enter a port,
they can be lightened by discharging part of their cargo into smaller
tankers lying a few miles off shore.[2] The port authority concerned will

[1] At Lisbon, in Portugal, a consortium of Swedish, Dutch, and Portuguese companies
have (September 1969) announced a venture to construct a dry dock for 500,000 d.w.t.
tankers with provision for expansion.
[2] Technical limitations for large tankers are shown by the fact that in 1968 tankers
over 50,000 d.w.t. used fifty-seven loading ports whilst vessels over 200,000 d.w.t. used
only four. The latter tonnage is considered to be the most economical of the range of
mammoth tankers.

be expected to give facilities for this either within estuarial waters within their control or along the coast and near to the port. If the bulk vessel is employed on a shuttle service, for the running of which the total annual requirements of material have been calculated, then the size of the vessel can be kept down to a tonnage which, multiplied by the practical number of voyages, will enable this quantity to be handled each year.[1]

A feature that, although not new, has never before been so clearly demonstrated in the shipment of cargo, is the effect of size on operating costs. Going back to the principle that the ship consists of a propelling unit linked with a carrying unit, it is obvious that whilst the former can be kept fairly constant in size, the latter can expand to the limit of what is found to be practical. If, for instance, the problem is to haul 50 million gallons of oil from the Persian Gulf to a western European port, this could be done in three tankers, each of some 66,700 d.w.t. Alternatively, it could be accomplished in one tanker of 190,000 d.w.t. Whatever the size of the ship, the most expensive part must always be present—[2]the electronic and navigational equipment, the crew's quarters, and the engines. Substantially the cost of equipping a ship with these and other essential parts does not depend on her size. The thirty men who operate the smaller tanker can also operate the larger one, which, incidentally, uses very little more fuel to carry three times the load at a very slightly lower speed. It is not surprising that the larger tanker, too big to use the Suez Canal, can transport oil from the Persian Gulf to Europe for 10s. (50p) a ton cheaper than can a smaller vessel when able to use the Canal and thus making the voyage 4000 miles shorter. There is, therefore, little attraction in ships less than the 200,000 d.w.t. size. If the Canal is to be dredged so that it will be able to take the larger ships in ballast, then, to pay for this work, canal dues will have to be raised. This will make the route, already the first casualty in Middle East politics, even less attractive.

Discussion following the 1967 closing of the canal has included a suggestion to lay a 42-inch pipeline, capable of carrying 50 million tons of oil a year, from Suez to Port Said. Oil for European markets would be discharged at the southern terminus of the pipeline from tankers which are

[1] The owners must, however, consider the possibility, however remote, of the mammoth ship for whatever reason becoming a casualty. If this happened would there be a ship of similar size available for charter? If not, then the whole logistic pattern, built up around the super-ship, would have to be reorganized at short notice to operate with whatever ships were available.

[2] The articulated ship attempts to overcome this.

envisaged to be of the incredible size of one million d.w.t. The oil would be reloaded at the northern end of the canal on to smaller tankers that could ship direct to European refineries. This is, indeed, to take advantage of the economy to be found in large cargoes. It is a far cry from the expensive transhipment of general cargo in small quantities and on camel-back by the overland route which operated successfully from 1837 across the Suez isthmus until the opening of the Suez Canal in 1869.

As a final word on size it is admitted that the idea of a 500,000 d.w.t. tanker is a challenging one to the industry, with its promise of a freight cost on a 10,000-mile voyage of just under £1 a ton. The challenge lies also in a whole range of tricky operational, navigational, and handling problems that demonstrate how impossible it is to take any ship problem in isolation from shippers, receivers, and the ports. The practice of discharging part cargoes from the mammoths into small tankers near to the ports, entry into which would be simple, will figure largely in the future.

In these days of automation and computers it is refreshing to find the human element sticking out like a sore thumb into calculations that seem to many to defy nature. Whilst the vessel is at sea the crew are doing their duty. This is what they are there for and what they are paid to do. As a giant tanker makes her 17-day journey from Japan to Kuwait there is the frustration of passing many exotic places without the opportunity of going ashore. With a crew of officers and men of not more than thirty-two it is not difficult for loneliness and boredom to set in and a general melancholy that has already been expressed as "the tanker sickness". Where there is complete dedication to the job and a national pride in participating in a technical achievement, of which each man can feel he is playing a part, added to the paternalistic loyalty to be found in Japanese shipping circles, then the conditions will not become so marked. It is easy, however, to see that particular attention will have to be paid to the crew problem of the non-stop voyage of the mammoth tanker, particularly when this is combined with the scanty leisure enjoyed with the hurried turnround at each port. Some confidence is felt that progress may lie in recent agreements to replace "able seamen" by "operators". This will be done by the breaking down of the rigid barriers that have always separated engine and deck crews. The crew member will find variety in becoming a general-purpose engineer.

Ore is a commodity that has taken advantage of the lower transport costs per ton that flow from the bigger carrying vessel. It is estimated that the United Kingdom demand for imported iron ore will by the mid 1970s have risen from 15 to 22 million tons. There is, however, with ore the problem of finding suitable ports for discharge, and the question of draught is important (Fig. 11). Until recently a maximum loaded draught of 42 ft would have meant a cargo of certainly not more than 65,000 tons, but by increasing the beam and, to a lesser degree, the length, a ship of this draught will now carry up to 80,000 tons. There is the prospect that the Japanese ore ports will be able to take ships of 100,000 tons (about 47-ft draught), and that Port Talbot in South Wales may berth carriers up to

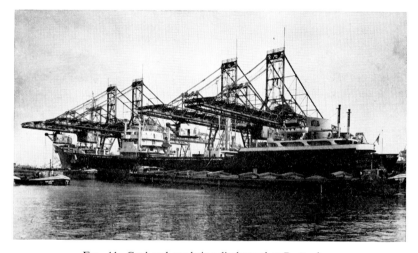

FIG. 11. Coal and ore being discharged at Rotterdam.

150,000 d.w.t. Discharge is done by out-size grabs each with a capacity of 12½ tons; each of the five transporter–unloaders can discharge ore in this way to conveyor berths at a rate of 500 tons per hour.[1]

As part of the shipping revolution that is changing the types, the shapes and the purposes of ships, is the new OBO carrier. This is short for oil, bulk, and ore, and it is the intention to avoid the wasteful period ore-carriers spend in ballast. The OBO vessel can be filled with oil for one voyage, later changing her cargo to ore or grain.

[1] As a sidelight on the carrying of ores in bulk, the *David P. Reynolds*, 47,000 d.w.t., was launched at Hamburg in the summer of 1969 to carry aluminium ore. A foundry is to be built by 1972 within the port area, and this will employ 1200 people.

General

In the very early ferry ships, loading of vehicles was supervised by stevedores. Their presence was a relic of the days when each car had to be slung, often before the eyes of the apprehensive owner, and taken on board very much as a set of general cargo. It was quickly realized that on a ferry only token supervision was necessary. Each item of cargo is fully mobile and has a co-operative driver who supplies the petrol to drive the car and the labour to place it on the spot indicated by the ship. At the end of the voyage the same driver, hitherto the shipper, now becomes the receiver. Completely under his charge and at his expense, the ship's cargo is unloaded in so short a time that ferries from Southampton to Cherbourg—a longish voyage for Channel vessels—can make three turnrounds daily during the season.

Other loads on wheels were quick to take advantage of the door-to-door principle. Heavy packages and containers can be lifted from the carrying vehicle by straddle carriers and transferred into the hold of the ferry. With a heavy duty equipment of this kind a fully loaded transport non-passenger ferry vessel can be discharged and loaded (the cargo including seventy-five trailers, containers, and other large packages) in 4 hours.

Single-pull Hatches

A minor improvement, but one that makes a daily contribution to ship turnround, is the single-pull system of hatch covers. Until this was invented in the late 1950s, the design of hatch coverings had hardly altered since the days of sail. It was not conceivable that cargo could be protected otherwise than by high coamings on to which were fitted small, wooden hatches,[1] the whole being covered by triple tarpaulins made secure by being wedged into cleats. This elaborate defence against weather took time and labour to assemble and to take apart. This had to be done at the beginning and at the end of each working period, and again when rain threatened. The single-pull hatch assembly made possible much larger openings in the deck, also produced coverings that were flush, not only on the top deck but also in the 'tween decks. This was important because the obstacles to using forklift trucks on all the decks was now removed.

---

[1] To make them easily handlable, one shipping line had hatch covers so small that they were colloquially known as "dominoes".

Voyage Time and Time Spent in Ports

After the Second World War ship designers concentrated on increasing the speed of cargo ships. A damper on their efforts was the knowledge that time gained at sea at considerable constructional expense could only too easily be lost by the currently inefficient cargo-handling methods. It would be better, knowledgeable shipowners thought, to attack the very much more difficult problems that were delaying ship turnround and to leave the voyage time until the time taken in port had been reduced from the appalling figure of 235 days in each year. Such were conditions in 1950; there is no doubt that the figure for 1969 would show improvement as a result of the great strides in cargo-handling methods of the last two decades.[1] There is now felt to be a need for vessels that would bridge the gap between the 25-knot container ship and the 400-knot air freighter, particularly for operation on the North Atlantic. Experiments on the "container air bubble" (CAB) principle would, it is claimed, be very worth while.[2]

Coastal Shipping

Contrary to opinion in some quarters, the carriage of goods by coastal and near-continental lines has not been obliterated in British shipping circles by containers, road traffic, or bulk vessels. Not only are coal cargoes foreseen for several years, but the demands of the building and construction trades call for movement of large quantities of stone, slag, and cement—in fact a low-value high-capacity cargo. Irish potatoes can also be included in this category as well as participation in the trans-shipment of optional cargoes discharged at continental ports; the establishment of refineries in the United Kingdom has produced a big demand for the coastwise shipment of specialized petroleum products.

Conclusion

Progress in the design and building of ships has been mainly in the direction of providing facilities for carrying and for handling of special cargo. It has become noticeable in many major ports that although the modern cargo liner continues to supply the balance of imported general

[1] The incidence of labour stoppages cannot be ignored.
[2] The CAB ship would have a size of 5000 d.w.t. with a suggested propulsion system of eight marine gas turbines each developing 25,000 b.h.p. It is considered possible to build ships of this kind for a 100-knot cargo service across the North Atlantic within 10 years.

cargo, the arrival of a new vessel designed entirely for the deep-sea package, or break-bulk trade, is becoming a rare event.

The present trend can be summed up as providing a role for the ship which far exceeds that of a mere carrier which accepted cargo in whatever quantity and condition it suited the shipper to present it. The concept of the container would collapse were the ship's interest in her cargo to commence, as hitherto, at the ship's rail and to end, similarly, at the port of destination. The container ship is in fact the triumph of the idea of through transportation for general cargo. This, added to the development of large ships for liquids and for bulk cargoes, is making large sections of the world's shipping obsolescent. It is no gradual process, like the change-over from sail to steam that took half a century to make an impression: it is a swift and dramatic change that is full of challenge to shipowners. It has brought many casualties to the accepted ideas that have held sway for centuries. A major casualty has been, and will continue to be, the demand for dock labour; this will be more fully treated in a later chapter. It is enough here to say that throughout the changing story of ship development, whether it be the birth of the container ship or the adoption of single-pull hatches, there runs the single principle of a declining need for the manual handling of cargo—a need that has supported generations of port workers.

Additional Notes

Chapter 3, page 37, par. 2. Roll-on ships. Built for service between Genoa and Palermo, the *Freccia Rossa* and her sister ship have three stern doors to speed movement of vehicles.

Page 41, par. 2. Pusher ships. The proposed U.S. tug-barge combination has a tug positioned inside a special "slot" at the barge's stern.

Page 45, par. 2. Nuclear-powered ships. The first of these, the *Savannah*, has been laid up as uneconomic.

Page 52, par. 1. Voyage time. Under development in the U.S. is the TRISEC ship with a proposed speed of 50 knots.

CHAPTER 4

THE CARGO

Introduction

1945 is, once more, a convenient date to commence tracing the explosive development in the modernizing of cargo in its presentation for shipment and in its handling by the ship and by the port operator on the quay. There is a single thread which runs through this story—the search for the larger cargo unit. Although it can be expressed in so few words, the process has been and continues to be—for it will never finish—a complex study in which the results have, in the main, been very rewarding. From that earliest attempt at unitized cargo, leaving the sling on the set at shipment,[1] through the many stages of pallets and containers to shipment in bulk, the largest possible cargo unit has been achieved. In the immediate wake of these developments has been the inescapable shadow—the reduction in the demand for labour to handle cargo. Although this has been felt in the early and the late stages of transportation, it is the intermediate handling at the ports where redundancy has been most marked.

Changed Methods in Packing Cargo

These have been legion, and hardly a staple commodity but has been examined with the intention of altering conventional forms of packaging. Nothing has been sacred; prejudices, traditions, and customs of the port have gone overboard, and the net result has been not—as predicted—to kill a trade but to make the handling of a major import more economic.

WINE

No form of cargo over the last 1000 years has been treated with more reverence than wine. Carried in casks, almost the earliest form of container (they were used by the Babylonians), handled with the greatest care, and

---

[1] Bags of soda ash have been shipped palletized and kept in position with a cheap disposable cargo sling.

requiring the skilled attention of a cooper before they could be moved from the ship's hold, all these unwritten laws had supposedly to be obeyed for the wine to be in good condition on arrival. A faster, cheaper, and more efficient method was demanded to meet the increasing imports of moderately priced wines that followed the Second World War. Shipment in large steel tanks which had been treated with a wine-resistant composition followed early experiments with glass-lined containers and with none of the disastrous results predicted either to the flavour or taste of the wine. Whilst the more expensive blends continued to be shipped in casks, wine in increasing quantities from Spain, Italy, Portugal, and Cyprus came in bulk. Pumping the wine out from the ship's tanks to glass-fibre-lined vats in the shore installation presented little difficulty and is done at the rate of 3000 gallons per hour per pump (Fig. 12). Neither was there difficulty

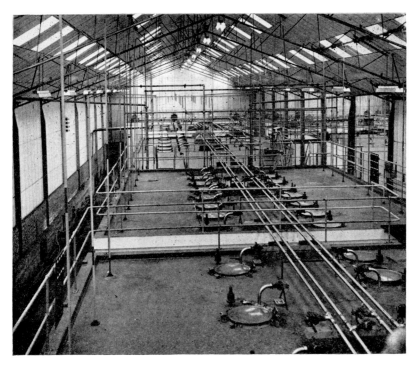

FIG. 12. Bulk wine installation, West India Dock, London.
(By courtesy of PLA.)

in delivery to bulk road carriers. In the port of London the initial storage capacity for wine in bulk, fixed at 380,000 gallons, is expected to reach one million gallons as more types of wine prove suitable for handling in this way. The quantity that will pass through shore installations will increase as importers turn over from cellar storage to bulk. On a minor note, grape-juice concentrate, used in the manufacture of wines within the United Kingdom is being imported from the Argentine in containers. Whisky, a major United Kingdom export, will also be carried in stainless-steel container tanks, each with a capacity of 4700 imperial gallons.

TIMBER

In the 1820s, softwood timber was first imported in cut form (deals, boards, and battens) in place of the round logs that had hitherto been cut at the port of destination. Ship space was saved and the amount of timber imported increased as the Victorian building boom made further inroads on European and American forests.[1] For nearly a century and a half the drawbacks of handling timber in loose condition were accepted. For the tight stowage achieved in the ship, the price had to be paid at the discharging port. Each piece had to be handled in the making up of the set—the only unit load known in the industry, and that with a life at the most of a few minutes. Either the set was shot loose into a barge or the sling pulled and the contents dumped on the quay under plumb of the ship's gear. Discharge was slow, so slow that demurrage on the ship was regarded as inevitable, and the holder of each bill of lading had to make his contribution to a demurrage fund. After the ship had left the quay, the tedious job of sorting to dimensions the many thousand loose pieces and conveying these, a few at a time, on the shoulders of deal porters, to a final stowage on open ground or in a shed adjacent to the berth, was tackled. With the coming of mechanization in the early 1950s, the process was speeded up in the piling stages. Softwood handling was seasonal owing to the icing-up of many of the loading ports. It was possible neither to predict nor to regulate arrivals; ports became, in the event, congested, with newly arrived ships waiting in the stream for a berth on which it was not uncommon to see the cargo of the later ship dumped ashore on top of the remains of an earlier cargo that had been only partially removed for piling. Craft loaded with softwood took many days to discharge; many wharves had no cranes and each piece had to be "walked" out by dealporters. As the season

[1] United Kingdom imports of 1968 were, softwood—1,932,361 standards.

advanced, congestion of craft impeded other work in the docks; shortage of craft slowed down discharge already commenced (Fig. 13). After the trade had recovered from the shortage of timber caused by the Second World War, imports into the United Kingdom ports rose to over 250 million pieces annually. It was estimated that from the time of shipment until use on a building site, each piece might be handled ten or a dozen times. No industry could show such wasteful methods of handling, and

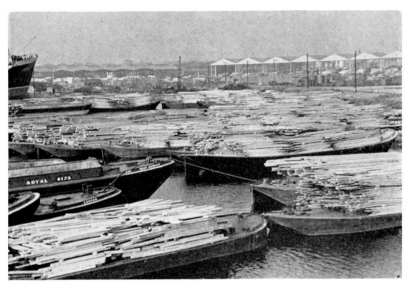

FIG. 13. Loose softwood in barges waiting to leave the Port of London. The heavy stocks of loose timber piled in the sheds and in the open, at the rear, illustrate conditions before the coming of packaged timber. (By courtesy of PLA.)

these included the large quantity that annually was lost overboard as pieces slipped out of sets during discharge or were bumped off laden barges as they bored their way through the congested dock water. No other industry accepted for so long conditions such as these with complacency, nor discovered so many reasons why changes should be resisted. The capital loss caused by the delay, often of months, before bills of lading could be brought to account and claims for shortage settled, apart from the cost of tallying (a process often of dubious value), was all reflected in the price of timber and, eventually, in the cost of the houses built. Speed of dispatch was not aided by the poor quality of the gear operated by many

T.E.P.—C

timber carriers nor by the frequency with which they arrived with ponderous deck cargoes which had shifted during the voyage, giving the vessel a dangerous list. Altogether, for a century or more, softwood imports were synonymous with poor dispatch, delays, and irritating shortages. The industry was overdue for modernization.

This was done by applying the principle of the unit load. In place of the single piece came the package in which about 100 pieces, all of the same size, were strapped together. All the pieces within the package were, in fact, similar in length, width, and thickness. Sorted prior to banding and shipment, the identity of the package was maintained during the voyage, the discharge, the removal from the ship and the delivery to barge, and to the final stowage ground alongside the berth. The immediate advantage of the packaged timber traffic, which intruded in 1958 into the old-world methods of the industry, insisted on being noticed. Timber in this form could now be taken from the ship's side and placed into final stowage within not months but minutes; the importer could have his piling account the next day and with no shortages that had to be identified from the specification and then argued about with the underwriter.

From the sailing ships that lingered in the softwood trade until the First World War, discharged often by their own not very efficient crews, and the small vessels of low capability that crossed the North Sea until after the Second World War, timber ships have become larger and speedier and therefore more expensive to run. From British Columbia, with its exports encroaching on European sources, ships have reached 17,000 g.r.t. It would be unthinkable for a ship of this size to struggle with loading and discharging a cargo of loose timber. Also they are too big for many of the smaller and old-fashioned docks where a primitive traffic in loose timber still lingers.[1] New methods had to be devised; deep-water berths with ample quay space made it economic to land the entire cargo and subsequently to deliver to craft the overside portion. From the original size of a package weighing about 1 ton, the unit has now reached a normal weight of 3 tons.[2] The handling of these has been made possible by installing quay cranes to supplement the ship's gear, providing side-lifting fork-

[1] The m.v. *Kotlasles* made, in the autumn of 1969, three voyages carrying packaged timber, from Archangel to London. The ship was successfully discharged at the special berth for packaged timber at Tilbury Dock; considerable increase in the shipment in packaged form, from Russia to United Kingdom ports, will result from this experiment.

[2] Softwood is now being shipped from British Columbia, in packaged form, in units each of 15 tons, shipped as deck cargo.

lift trucks for receiving and running the packages away from the ship's side, and heavier forklift trucks of a normal design for piling the bills of lading that remain in store. The most modern carriers built for the packaged timber trade carry their own cranes which have a capacity of 18 tons and straddle the ship's deck so that the delivery of the cargo is possible both ashore and into craft.

A quay shed is a useful asset on a berth of this kind, and will house parcels of plywood, liner boards, paper, etc., that accompany cargoes of softwood. Refinements such as specially designed spreaders and very up-to-date labour arrangements, to which reference will be made in a later chapter, have contributed to outputs that can be described as phenomenal. They are entirely outside the comprehension of port operators technically efficient at operating the conventional and tedious methods in use for so many years on loose timber. A satisfactory output on this kind of cargo would have been 1000 tons a day. With the packaged type, 4000 tons is aimed at; deliveries from the berth to lorry have reached 2000 tons a day. It is not surprising that a conservative estimate places the reduction in port handling costs at £10 a standard. This is apart from the savings in freight, insurance, and administrative expenses incurred by the importer; the cheaper cost to the barge or to the lorry owner in turnround time is significant. Demurrage both of the ship and the craft is now an old, unhappy memory of past inefficiency.

A study by the Timber Research and Development Association (TRADA) has helped in gaining acceptance by the trade of the many radical changes necessary; standardization of sizes among other problems has been tackled. So successful has packaging become that the docks that are built for handling pieces of softwood have now only a precarious future. From the west coast of Africa, cut hardwood lumber is now being shipped in pre-sorted and packaged form. This is an industry where modernization presents many problems, but the prizes already secured by their softwood colleagues dangle before the eyes of the hardwood importers.

SUGAR

The very important change from sugar imported in bags to sugar imported in bulk has been mentioned already. Once a major source of employment for dock workers, the handling by grabs from bulk to shore conveyors has almost taken this staple import out of the range of general cargo work.

Sundry Cargoes

It is difficult to think of any homogeneous imports of any size that have not been affected by the urge to find a larger basic unit: only a few can be quoted here.

MEAT

Since the first import of chilled and refrigerated meat into the United Kingdom in the latter part of the last century, the general principle of making up sides and carcasses into sets has been followed. Some improvement in dispatch has been made recently by packing meat into cartons, and this has enabled pocket elevators to be lowered into the holds with the cargo fed to the boot of the elevator by small portable belt conveyors.[1] The excessive sorting to marks and qualities demanded by the very many receivers that form the meat trade has for years defeated attempts to handle this type of cargo mechanically. Now the sorting ashore is being done on conveyors, and the destination of each cargo unit is controlled by a computer. As all parts of the landing and delivery system are enclosed, work is done independently of weather conditions; rain, which damaged frozen meat, always stopped work. Some of the earliest attempts to provide protection for cargo during wet weather were prompted by the vulnerability of frozen and chilled meat.

To avoid delays and congestion with lorries applying for meat, a lorry control park with marshalling and calling up arrangements is operated. Experience with this new method of handling meat, first tried out at Bluff in New Zealand, has revealed advantages not all of which were foreseen at its inception. There is the very considerable step-up in output, with the turnround of the ship expedited and delays to lorries cut considerably. Manual handling has been reduced and with it damage to the cargo. The heavy cost of manual tallying and of sorting by staff has been cut and accuracy has been obtained. The equipment provided for meat can also be used for the fast discharge, including sorting and tallying, of com-

[1] A new packaging process threatened (July 1969) to do away with the traditional overhead rail-handling methods in refrigerated holds of ships. Freshly cut and boned meat is placed in bags made of a moisture, gas, and bacteria proof film; loss from drip and evaporation is eliminated and the meat can be stored at chill temperatures for up to 6 weeks. The bags are transported in easily handled plastic crates weighing about 60 lb. A space saving over the hanging of hinds and fores in the hold is estimated at 500 per cent.

modities such as butter and fruit. Cargo in cartons or boxes lends itself to handling by this means.

GRAIN

Since the exploitation of the American Prairies in the 1880s grain in bulk has been a familiar sight in the ports of importing countries. After a slow start, by bagging the loose grain by hand, the bucket elevator was brought into use to be followed in the early years of the present century by the suction machine. Since the introduction of this very useful plant (it can also be used for discharging cotton seed and copra in bulk), progress has been concentrated on removing obstacles to fast discharge. With the very modern installations at Amsterdam and London, to mention two ports alone, shore silos have been increased in capacity so that the discharge of a newly arrived ship does not have to wait on the clearance of the grain terminal. The problem of work slowing down as the ceiling of the ship's hold is reached has been tackled, as has that of delays to powerful elevators caused by the frequent shuffling of small capacity craft. Permanently fixed shore elevators have long been part of the port pattern. A recent improvement allows the suction plant to travel along a rail track 18 ft wide, running parallel with the quay. Each of these two legs has a capacity of 200 tons per hour, and they work into a silo that holds 25,000 tons. As the track runs for 500 ft (the working length of a 10,000 d.w.t. ship), the twin elevators can be made to plumb any of the holds.

As an illustration of the trend with an industry that made increasing use of ports, in the early days grain was delivered to receivers in bags. This suited the convenience of millers, but it seriously delayed the discharge of the ship. After the Second World War, as more receivers equipped their premises with suction plant, port authorities discouraged bagging of grain ex-ship, even to the extent of not incorporating these facilities in new machines that were built. Where bagging has still to be done, it has been found more economical and far more speedy than bagging loose grain on the quay (a practice still to be found in some ports) for grain to be discharged in bulk into rail wagons. These are hauled to a depot outside the port area where bagging can be done at much lower labour costs. The quay is left clear for continuous discharge.

An auxiliary but very useful piece of plant is the portable pneumatic elevator (Fig. 14). As it weighs only 5 tons it can be worked from the deck of a ship to pour grain into a barge or it can, working from the quay, suck grain from a barge and deliver it to road or rail conveyance. It does, in fact, provide the answer to those receivers who still insist on having their parcels of grain delivered ex-ship or ex-silo in bags. As some types have been constructed as self-propelled units, their usefulness has been very much extended.

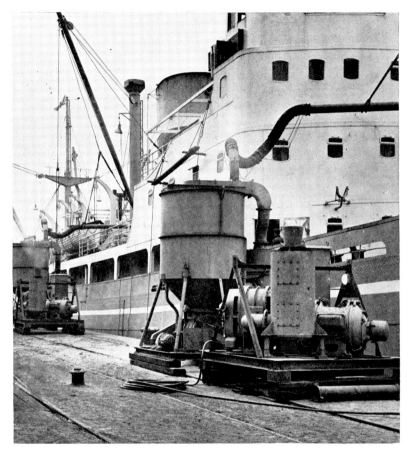

FIG. 14. Mobile grain elevators operating from the quay.
(By courtesy of Simon Engineering Ltd.)

APPLES

As the growing of fresh fruit for export developed, shippers continued to cling to customs that had originated with the traffic and which progressively hindered its expansion. It was natural that every grower should take pride in decorating the few cases of apples he produced, with elaborate markings which, whilst they publicized his venture, confused the docker and made the sorting in the dock shed of a complete shipload an extremely involved and slow process. Shed space, manual labour, and staff supervision were uneconomically employed in maintaining what must have been one of the most wasteful of all "customs of the port". Now apples from Tasmania have been imported in large wooden bins weighing half a ton and whose contents are equivalent to twenty-five boxes. As the contents are of the one quality and size, these large bins can be taken direct from the ship for retail distribution.

TOMATOES, VEGETABLES, ETC.

As with apples so with tomatoes and vegetables, although the load here consists of palletized baskets made up into a cargo unit that can be delivered direct from the wharf to the customer. Citrus fruit is already being handled in this way with a quicker turnround of land transport at the port of loading, reduced manual gangs at both terminals, and elimination of much sorting before delivery. Where citrus fruit has not been palletized, the use of code systems to replace individual markings for each size and quality has reduced the time and labour required for sorting many thousand boxes in the dock shed. With produce that is fighting the menace of decreased consumption and competition from new sources, attention is being paid to expanding the processed market both in grapefruit and orange juice.

BANANAS

Bananas are another fruit grown and shipped under the threat of new growing areas. Over-production has led to many improvements since the 1920s when stems of bananas were imported, each packed in a thin plywood cylinder. In 1929 they arrived "naked", and a sizeable quantity from each shipment was expected to reach port in an overripe or damaged condition. During the last few years much progress has been made in selecting only the prime hands for export. These are packed in standard sized cartons to the exclusion of fruit of poorer quality and the heavy and useless stems. Attention has also been given to shipment of unit loads of cartons on pallets; this method would, it is thought, eliminate delay to discharge and damage to the fruit. Bananas in cartons, even if not palletized, would be a suitable cargo for handling by the computerized meat conveyor described earlier (Fig. 15).

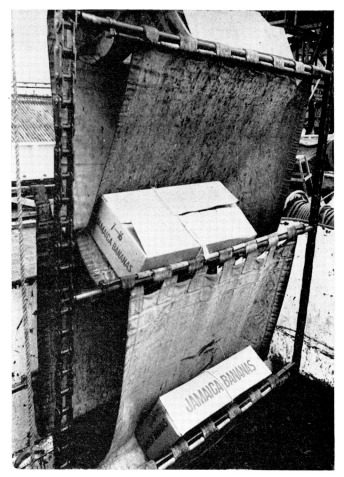

FIG. 15. Bananas in cartons being discharged on an elevator designed for handling bananas in stems. (By courtesy of PLA.)

MOLASSES, EDIBLE FATS, ETC.

A valuable byproduct of the sugar industry is molasses. Until the Second World War many tons of this sticky liquid were shipped in iron drums;

small ventilating holes were left open in each, with the result that handling at discharge was a slow and dirty business which attracted extra payment for labour. For some years now the liquid has been shipped in bulk in ship's tanks and pumped out direct to terminals (there is one at Hull and another at Liverpool) from which it is delivered to bulk lorries for road destinations. Edible fats have also been melted down to be pumped into tank stowage on the carrying vessel.

CARBON BLACK

To say that carbon black in bags had the greatest nuisance value per ton of any imported cargo would not have been contradicted by any port operator called upon regularly to handle this essential element in tyre manufacture. Baths on the spot and changes of clothing had to be provided, apart from the high cost of piecework handling. Now specially designed containers have been invented with the contents of which the dockers are not directly concerned.

SULPHUR AND POTASH

Sulphur was always carried in lump- and powder-form and was a dusty and objectionable cargo discharged by grabs or, earlier still, in canvas nets. There was always the risk of fire from friction; contamination from foreign objects was difficult to avoid. For the past 10 years the United States have shipped sulphur in liquid form, and this practice has now been extended to Europe. A centre for the reception and for the distribution of liquid sulphur to consignees on the Continent has been built at Rotterdam. Should there be an interruption in the supply of liquid sulphur, the centre is capable of receiving and storing it as a solid and, subsequently, liquefying it.[1] Potash is another commodity that requires stock piling because the chemical industry has to be able to rely on a constant supply. Due to the fine and dusty nature of potash, chutes and conveyors used at discharge and stockpiling have to be specially constructed and roofed, whilst the plant has to be guarded against corrosion and the potash from moisture.[2] A port such as Rotterdam that is centrally situated to act as a distribution

[1] Bulk sulphur is now (July 1970) imported into both London and Immingham.
[2] The Tees and Hartlepool Port Authority have (June 1969) installed a covered shiploader for bulk cargoes. It consists of a bulk loading conveyor which will receive bulk cargo from road vehicles and discharge it into the ship's hold without exposing it to the weather.

centre to a major industrial hinterland will attract developments such as the above. Borax and aluminia are among other chemicals now imported in bulk and which lend themselves to processing at installations served directly from the carrying vessel.

NEWSPRINT

One of the most vulnerable of all imports was newsprint. Its discharge, and subsequent handling and delivery from the dock shed, was a slow and

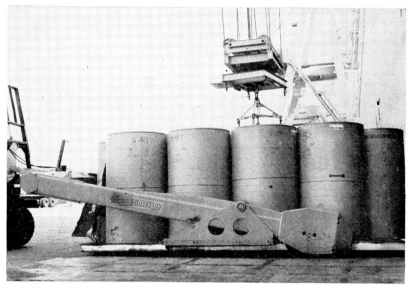

FIG. 16. Rolls of paper discharged by special gear at Canadian Transport (Terminals Ltd.) berth at Tilbury Dock, London. (By courtesy of PLA.)

tedious process that had to be stopped in bad weather. Now there are means of unitizing this cargo when carried on modern vessels built specially for this traffic. The ship has two gantry cranes each capable of lifting 20 tons. An electrically operated clamp dispenses with manual handling and can lift sixty-four bales of paper weighing 14 tons at a time; complete protection from weather is also provided (Fig. 16).

MOTOR-CARS

Few exports have passed through more teething troubles than unpacked cars. Vulnerable at all points to damage and to rough usage, they were expected to arrive overseas in showroom condition. After experimenting in providing false timber decks to general-cargo ships and to enclosing each car in a tubular scaffolding cage, stowed in the open-deck type of bulk carrier, reliance is now being placed on the "knocked down" condition; here vehicles are exported in pieces and reassembled in factories in the importing country. By this means an awkward export, composed very largely of air spaces and odd-shaped pieces of metal, can be economically packed in parts of similar size, the whole consisting of a number of large cargo units which, virtually, are a form of container. Thirty completely knocked down Land Rovers can be packed into two standard sized containers each 20 ft by 8 ft by 8 ft for shipment to Australia.

RICE

This very fine commodity has always called for particularly careful handling when shipped in bags. With a cargo that "ran" very easily, stevedores' hooks were forbidden in stowage and breaking out; rain interfered with loading. There are now vessels of 10,000 d.w.t. carrying 500,000 bushels of rice in bulk, built specially for this commodity. The traffic demands special storage facilities ashore, including silos similar to those in use for bulk grain. At the port of loading, conveyors take the rice directly into the ship's holds at a rate of 600 tons per hour.

CEMENT

A familiar bag cargo, particularly in the Thames Estuary, cement in bags was suitable for the bottom stowage of ships. A new system that relies largely on belt conveyors is now in use for handling cement in bulk form. The plant has been designed to cope with the bulk loading of ships or of craft for coastwise shipment. Complete protection from weather and damp is given, and the cement—after passing through a junction house on the quay—is discharged through two telescopic chutes into the hold of the waiting ship. An electronic weigher records not only a running total of the weight of the cement delivered to the jetty, but automatically cuts off the feed when the amount required has been delivered. Compared with the conventional loading in bags, this method has made many economies, not the least being the great reduction from the standard ship gangs to the few men needed to control the machinery. Inter-state transportation of cement in bulk is done in Australia by bringing the cement in trains made up of 45-ton automatic dump wagons operating a 24-hour-a-day service.

It is shipped by the n.v. *Burwah*, fitted with machinery that allows discharge of her 3000 ton cargo at a rate of 500 tons per hour.

Where conditions prevent shipment of cement in bulk improvement over the crane method has been made by using a spiral chute for transferring the bags from the jetty to the hold. As the feed belts and the telescopic belt are covered by sheet metal, they are rainproof. Two men are sufficient to stow the bags in the hold of the ship.

CHINA CLAY

A minor but valuable bulk export from Great Britain is china clay. The powdered clay is compressed into blocks each weighing 25 kg. Each block is wrapped in paper; forty are interlocked and strapped together to form a self-palletized load which, singly or in pairs, can be lifted and conveyed by forklift truck. Each unit weighs 1 ton and occupies 45 per cent less room than the equivalent weight in bags.

COPRA

Reference has already been made to the use of suction machines for discharging copra in bulk. Although they have been so employed for many years, output has been poor—eight men in the hold of a ship would not induce more than 30 tons per hour to pass along the suction pipes. After a long sea voyage from the Far East, the copra arrived with the shells in a solid mass. Each shell had to be loosened before it could be caught up in the air flow. Working with picks and shovels on this task in the confined conditions of the hold was an extremely unpleasant and unrewarding job.

Now a machine that will do this without damaging the skin of each shell has been brought into use. The principle involves a suction plant mounted on a pontoon but fitted with manipulative and other devices for loosening, which form part of the suction tube assembly. Provision is made to enable the hold to be plumbed all over; the presence of stanchions, coamings, and brackets does not interfere with the working of the two blades which, mounted spirally on the revolving suction nozzle, dislodge the compacted shells without causing any damage to them. A number of other improvements have been incorporated in this machine. The two installations built and in use at Rotterdam can both handle 150 tons per hour; only two men are needed to manipulate the pipes. These uniquely designed elevators have been found to be suitable for the discharge of heavy grains such as soya and maize meal, pellets, and other derivatives

Ballast Cargoes

A problem that faced the designers of very specialized heavy lifting sh'ps was the control of the ship's stability when a lift of, perhaps, 300 tons was being made from the wharf to the hold and vice versa. In these circumstances the list on the ship could not be allowed to exceed $12\frac{1}{2}$ degrees; a counter-list can be produced by cross-pumping from one tank to another. Whilst one purpose of the large tank accommodation is to carry fuel oil, a profitable cargo of vegetable oil and liquid tallow has been designed as part of the ballasting system.

Underwater Tank Storage

To help in solving problems of the modern super-tanker which cannot move into the comparatively shallow water of the inshore jetty, a project is in hand[1] for the building on the sea bed of the Persian Gulf, and at a depth of 160 ft, of a circular, dome-shaped storage tank, weighing some 15,000 tons, to hold 70,000 tons of crude oil. Vessels will be able to tie alongside the submerged tank and load the crude oil even under severe weather conditions. The tank is being designed to be self-submerging.

Handling Conditions in the Ship

Parallel with the progress made in simplifying the form in which cargo can be shipped, of which some examples have been given, has been the introduction of certain mechanical facilities within the ship. This has been accompanied by structural changes that have, in the case of flush deck-hatches, already mentioned, made possible the free movement of cargo-carrying trucks over the 'tween decks.

Cocoa, an export of prime importance to West Africa, was, until recently, handled in bags by entirely manual means (excluding the ships' derricks). It is now handled by mechanical equipment that includes the stacking of bags for an accumulated stockpile, the transfer of these to loading towers, and feeding them into the ships' holds. There is an ingenious method of spacing the bags as they pass along the horizontal conveyor at $4\frac{1}{2}$-second intervals and of ploughing bags to alternate outloaders; each of these can handle up to 50 tons an hour.

[1] In September 1969 the first man-made storage tank of this kind, the *Khazzan Dubai I*, was towed to its resting place in the Arabian Gulf, some 58 miles off Dubhai. It will store oil from the surrounding off-shore Fateh field.

In the early days of bulk cargo a major problem was the discharge of dry and often non-pulverulent materials. The struggles that took place with bulk sugar before the kangaroo crane, the grab, and the conveyor were installed, are now a matter of port history. Where the conditions are favourable, the small calf dozer has been found to be very effective and, as it can pick up a ton or more at a time, it is more economical than the filling of skips by manual labour.

Apart from the open-deck type of ship, already noticed, that added considerably to the area directly under plumb, another attempt to do away with the uneconomic horizontal movement of cargo in a ship's hold has arrived with the pallet deck vessel. The principle here is briefly, that unitized cargo can be stowed in the ship as easily as books can be placed on a shelf, but with the difference that the "shelf" can be brought forward so that each "book" can be placed in position from above. The vessel has four decks and each deck can be brought forward under plumb, loaded with palletized cargo, and returned to the wings; at discharge the process is reversed. In the absence of unitized cargo it is possible to load the decks with general cargo, but this is a slower process. An advantage of this method is that it does away almost entirely with broken stowage whilst making it possible to take out cargo at intermediate ports of call without the time and labour lost in re-stowing. As many cargo liners load and discharge at many ports, this is a simplification which should pay a good dividend.

Pallets that will achieve the much sought-after mobility of cargo have been produced by adapting the air cushion principle; they are known as "hoverpallets". They can be operated by one man who is able to move a large cargo unit over the deck or the ceiling of a ship.

In conclusion, a minor but long overdue improvement in cargo handling is worth mentioning. The pre-slinging of general cargo, particularly baled or packaged, has always been looked upon as the first and the most primitive form that the unit load could take. Progress in this obvious time-saver was prevented for some years because of the arguments over liability for injuries to workers and damage to the cargo; discharging stevedores were reluctant to use gear placed on board at the loading port. Now that this has been overcome, nylon webbing slings have been introduced on a major cargo liner service and the cost of handling sets of pre-slung bales and packages reduced by one-half. Steel rods in bundles have long been one of the most awkward of cargoes, both to load and to discharge; the process is simplified by pre-slinging. There is general agreement that in the years to come, when all cargo suitable has been packed into containers, there will still remain a large tonnage of general and special cargo that will resist the process. More and more attention will have to be paid to building this up into units by means of the pre-slung method.

This very brief survey of improvements in cargo handling since 1945 will fail in its object if it does not bring out the stark realism of the continuous and unending search made by shippers, shipping companies, and receivers of cargo for labour-saving methods. This will be examined in detail in a later chapter. Here, to take one commodity only, a glance at the changing conditions will illustrate the force of this overwhelming trend. Prior to the Second World War, sugar in bags was imported mainly through London and Liverpool. Some of the sugar went into store to await delivery. In 1938 the enclosed docks in London stored in their quayside warehouses 100,000 tons of bagged sugar. The labour needed to discharge this quantity ashore amounted to some 40,000 man hours. To house and to deliver this sugar would have brought the total up to 100,000 man hours of the port authority's labour alone. In 1949, when the first cargo of bulk sugar arrived in a United Kingdom port, 1,477,000 tons of sugar passed through Britain's two major ports. The great bulk of this was delivered to craft for the refineries. A very rough estimate of the labour required could be put at a million man hours. Against this permanent loss of manual effort can be placed the minute number of hours needed to transfer the cargoes of the bulk carriers from the ships' holds in to the refineries. The trade of the port of London was built up on sugar; the first enclosed dock, the West India Dock, opened there in 1802, was constructed with a 26-year monopoly of discharging all vessels arriving with sugar. Thirty years ago the disappearance of sugar in bags, as a staple import, would have been unthinkable. It is not alone now in being merely a fragrant memory.

Additional Notes

Chapter 4, page 58, par. 3. Softwood ships. The *Gimmeland*, 26,000 d.w.t., arrived Cardiff, with packaged timber, May 1970.

Page 59, par. 2. Output of softwood ships. The record is held (July 1970) by the *Norse Viking*, discharged at Tilbury Dock at a rate of 19·33 stdds per gang hour.

Page 70, par. 2. Unit loads. A Unit Load Council, with its H.Q. in Oslo, was established in May 1970 to promote the unit load concept.

Page 70, par. 3. Rolling cargo. The New Zealand CARGON system is based on rolling cargo instead of lifting units.

CHAPTER 5

MECHANIZATION

Introduction

Since 1945 several major trends have been discernible in the handling of cargo in the world's ports. They have tended to coalesce in the overall movement aimed at the quicker turnround of ships; it would not now be possible to separate them into their individual streams. Before 1939 the only recognizable trend was the ever-growing size of ships, and this was taking place more in the interests of passenger carrying than the movement of cargo.

The first and the most easily discernible of the post-war trends was the introduction of mechanical equipment into cargo handling. Tentatively brought in to cope with the appalling conditions of ports damaged during the Second World War, the early machines, the tractor and trailer and the mobile crane particularly, soon proved their worth. Where their use was possible, the early forklift trucks opened up a future for the port operator that took several years to define. This is a process by no means yet concluded. Having accepted the condition that dock work requires more sturdy appliances than does the factory or the depot, the special manufacture of equipment for ports became accepted. It has been uniformly successful and has been extended to such specialized areas as the 'tween decks and the holds of ships.

Over the centuries, dockworkers had generally known no other way of moving cargo than by muscle power aided by the wheeled handtruck and an explicit knowledge, and extensive application of the law of gravity.

How Men Work

The International Labour Organization, in a recent attempt to state the limiting load that a workman should be asked to handle, made three separate definitions of the major actions employed. Firstly, a man could, by imitating the jib of a crane, pick up a load at arms' length—28 lb was the limit here. Secondly, using the same method as the forklift truck, he could handle 156 lb. Whilst degrading himself to the level of a four-wheeled bogey he could carry, for a short distance, up to 500 lb on his back. Whether one agrees with the Labour Organization's conclusions or not, there can be no argument that the machine in each case does the job infinitely better. The machine has the great merit of not tiring. Piecework labour, when continued into overtime hours, has always been accompanied by a "loss of output" allowance, in recognition of Kipling's dictum "Morning never tries you till the afternoon". In passing it may be noted that every mechanical invention, with the exception of the wheel, has aimed to do the same operation as a human muscle but to do it better. Having regard to the cost of its upkeep and maintenance and in relation to its performance, using the human machine is the least economic way of getting work done.

Types of Equipment

The major tools of mechanization that have, after two decades of intense experiment, stood up to cargo handling are the forklift truck (Figs. 17 and 18), the mobile crane, the conveyor, and the tractor and trailer. No longer do port operators wonder if they should use this modern equipment; rather is their thinking directed to the type of machine that will most exactly satisfy their needs. Market research, intensive testing, and pooling of knowledge through international bodies such as ICHCA and ISO have tailored machines for special uses as well as introducing a variety of attachments to standard machines.

Benefits of Mechanization

Mechanization has driven many nails into the coffin of conventional dock working. Today the reception, storage, or delivery of cargo by old-established methods based on hand trucking and manual piling, would call for immediate investigation as to why this dark page of the past had not been turned. Mechanization has killed the bogey of distance; extra trucking—its cost a continuing loss to all port authorities and dock employers—no longer dominates the layout of port construction. For more than 100 years, storage facilities were based on the area that could be made available whether under cover or in the open. To extend this facility was possible only by manual piling, a costly device to which resort was only made under the threat of congestion. Today a tonnage of general cargo at least three times greater can be piled by forklift trucks on the same area

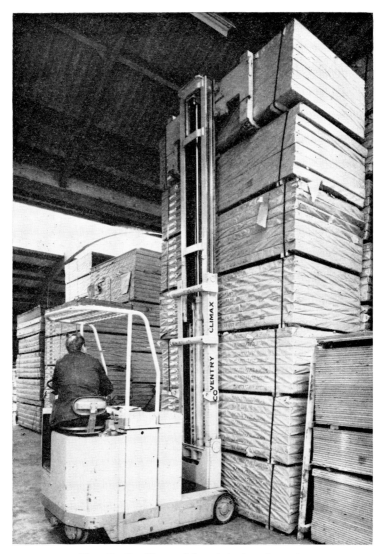

FIG. 17. Handling wall boards by forklift truck.
(By courtesy of Coventry Climax.)

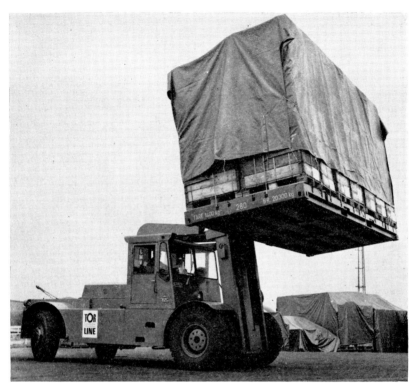

FIG. 18. 25 ton forklift truck handling a sheeted and unitized load for Tor
Line at Immingham Dock. (By courtesy of Tor Line.)

as that on which goods were hand pitched.[1] In producing a gang-hour
tonnage for mixed cargo far in excess of the 20–25 tons that was acceptable
in the inter-war period, the need for overtime working has been reduced.
The costs of tallying and supervision, with the larger tonnage handled,
have fallen steeply. A number of hidden costs, inseparable from the
leisurely working of pre-war days, have practically disappeared. The
machine can now, in the major number of instances, be taken to the job.
Overhead gantries, installed often for the handling of seasonal cargoes and
at very considerable cost for building and maintenance, have now been

[1] This is subject to delivery being taken from the top of the pile downwards and not
to picked numbers.

largely replaced by the mobile crane, brought in for the job and then taken away to work on the cargo of the next ship to arrive. By manipulation of this kind, machinery can now be used approaching the optimum of 312 days per annum (less periodical withdrawal for maintenance).

Present-day Mechanization

In the early post-war years a thorough investigation of much that had been accepted as normal dock work had to be made before the right machine for the job could be selected. Working operations were analysed. In the result it was found to be possible to separate the functions inherent in lifting a package and putting it down again in another place. Machines for making horizontal changes in the position of cargo units were set apart from those that could be used for vertical movement. Some machines were capable, it was found, of doing both jobs. In general there had to be a limitation in the use of each type of machine and a strict definition of the transporting unit as compared with the lifting equipment. For instance, although a mobile crane could pick up a load and travel with this, it was found to be wasteful so to employ it when the job belonged properly to a forklift truck. Again, the distance over which a forklift truck should be called upon to travel should not be allowed to approach that for which transport by tractor and trailer was the more suitable—and far cheaper— method. These were but a few of the earlier discoveries made by the pioneers of port mechanization on whose excellent and painstaking work later developments have been based.[1]

A Backward Look

Now that the teething troubles have been passed and a generation of port operators have come to regard mechanical handling as the normal approach to moving cargo, certain requisites for its success have become apparent. Firstly, the transfer from manual to mechanical handling can best be done under the auspices of the port authority. More and more the port authority tends to become the major port employer. For a successful change, capital, administrative, and executive ability are needed. With the best intentions a port authority cannot succeed if it has respon- sibility for part only of the dock process. If, for instance, the cargo it

---

[1] The conditions in which mechanical equipment was brought into use in port working are described in detail in Oram, *Cargo Handling and the Modern Port*, Chapter 4, Pergamon Press, 1965.

contracts to receive on the quay is discharged by a master stevedore of small status, it is of little use for the authority to mechanize the reception and removal when the discharge remains on conventional, i.e., manual lines. Modern methods have pertinently illustrated the time-wasting and irresponsible methods of cargo handling done against a background of fragmentary employers.

Responsibility of Other Parties

As well as complete co-operation among the employers on the wharf, a new conception of the duties of shipper and receiver has come to be accepted. In the early days of mechanization an appeal to shippers to present their cargo in a form that would help the port authority and the shipping company met with little response. Similarly, much of the good work done at the ship's side was undone at the delivery point; receivers saw little to their advantage in altering the methods at their depots to oblige a distant port authority. Before long a larger vision of cargo hand-ling projected itself; some obvious advantages became apparent. Export cargo sent to the port in unit loads could demand cheaper freight rates; port authorities were ready to reduce terminal charges.[1] The factory was able to clear its products more quickly; delays to road transport became a thing of the past as more and more ports adopted the drill for mechaniz-ing export cargo worked out by the pioneers in 1947. Similarly, by investing in a few forklift trucks the receiver could accept unit loads with quicker delivery at the docks and less delay at his depot as he learnt progressively to keep his unit intact further and further along the line.

Berth Conditions

The original acceptance of the revolutionary changes in berth design have now given place to a concentration on detailed improvement. The question, "Why should the lorry be discharged or loaded at the traditional spot outside the shed?" has led to the building of internal ramps so that the cargo can go directly from the pile, thus saving a transfer in detail. The pile in the shed is one large unit of cargo; the contents of the lorry are the next unit in line. It is sensible to cut out the hiatus when the cargo has, as hitherto, been broken down into small units in order to make the transfer

[1] A shipping company operating between Harwich and Copenhagen has (May 1969) cut cargo rates for unit loads, up to 40 per cent. Port authorities offer up to 30 per cent in reduction for unitized cargoes that can be shipped in the same form.

from pile to lorry. It is indicative of the approach that demands that cargo in the conventionally small manually handled unit can no longer be tolerated. In abolishing the single package, unit mechanization has been stretched—not yet to its limits—but a very long way from the time when the forklift truck was seen only as a complement to the hand-trucking gang. The respect now accorded to the large cargo unit has had its effect on labour, so important an aspect of recent changes that it will be dealt with in the following chapter.

Maintenance, etc.

Looking after the human machine was never accepted as the job of the employer. Dock plans of the 1880s reveal an almost 100 per cent concentration on work. Apart from a few crude latrines, amenities now generally provided and expected, such as canteens, wash places, cloak rooms, and medical and first-aid centres, were entirely absent. Similarly, with the new machines the best possible services for maintaining, repairing, and servicing—including the charging of electrically driven units—have been provided. Almost as difficult has been to enforce the principle that every unit must be withdrawn from use at its scheduled date, and that there can be no exception to this. "What I gained on the quay I lost in the garage", was the dire complaint of an early user. The lesson has been taken to heart, and not only is strict maintenance now enforced but commonsense rules for the safe working of the different machines have been instituted. The training of drivers, first introduced by forward-looking manufacturers as a sales gadget, has for long been accepted as the responsibility of the employer. Money spent on this has produced a good dividend. Standardized methods of training are now being talked about, and standardized controls for some types of machines are being actively considered.

Practices that Retard Mechanization

A machine works best when it is used on repetitive work; it does not like to be stopped while its driver thinks. The pattern of cargo handling accepted since the Industrial Revolution had come to include many practices introduced by the port authority or the employer as an inducement to shippers and receivers to bring their business to the port. Merchants were quick to realize that sampling, weighing, measuring, and similar practices done in the dock sheds would enable them to put their goods directly on the market. The dock shed could, in fact, be used temporarily as their own warehouse. The dock staff learnt to carry out opera-tions very proficiently that, properly, came within the province of the merchant. Whilst goods were manually handled, little delay was caused by the assistance given to the different trades that made use of the docks. The belief grew, and it is still widely held, that a prime function of the port authority is to give service to the users of the port. No one would quarrel with the principle. One has, however, to ask if it is justifiable to interfere with ship turnround so as to make it easier for a merchant to sell his goods. Alternatively, the question can be posed whether token weighing or sampling, done without interference with the major movement of the cargo, could not be accepted. Token examination of passengers' baggage at airports is now an accepted practice.

A new look has in fact been taken at many of the requirements of the national Customs. Protection of the revenue is the primary interest of this service. Its officers have been particularly co-operative in devising ways of continuing to do this whilst ensuring that the flow of cargo is not interrupted.

The Mobile Crane

Round this one item of equipment have revolved so many schemes for improving cargo handling that it demands a section to itself. The power-driven cranes that had replaced hand-operated cranes had always been fixed installations; they now became truly mobile.[1] The very limited movement possible to the tracked quay crane, whilst of value during ship work, rendered these important items of the working equipment prac-tically useless save for occasional barge work when the berth was not occupied by a ship. Here was capital lying idle and incurring maintenance costs, while vessels at another berth or in another dock were starved of crane power. After some care in designing, mobile cranes (Fig. 19) were produced for dock work, the primary object being to use them on seasonal traffic; as they could be adapted for use on general cargo, a reasonable prospect of all-the-year-round use was held out. The conception of a quay as a place where the processes of cargo handling can be done only with fixed or semi-fixed cranes is now passing. Similarly, dock warehouses have always been provided with wall cranes, if not for every loophole,

[1] As quay cranes were mounted on rails (of varying gauge) they were, strictly speaking, transportable units; they could be moved from hold to hold or fleeted along the quay to serve ships on adjacent berths. It was never claimed for them that they were mobile.

for each vertical series of delivery points. Again, these were used only as required. Once a warehouse had been filled with cargo in long-term storage, the expensive batteries of wall cranes would remain unused until the market

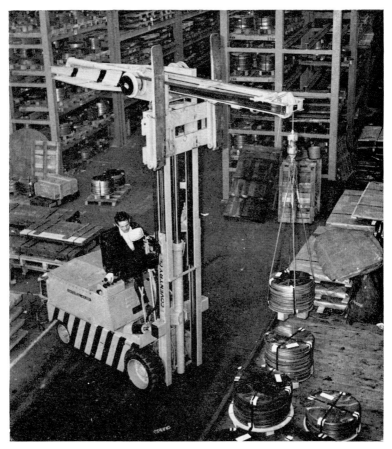

FIG. 19. Retractable overhead crane fitted to forklift truck.
(By courtesy of Coventry Climax.)

called for the delivery of the stored cargo. Meanwhile the periodic attention of the maintenance staff was necessary. Not only does the mobile
crane do the job as and when it is needed, but there are now types of forklift
trucks with out-size lifts that can take the goods away from the first floors

of warehouses. The old convention that ruled dockland for a century and more that the job must be taken to the machine has now given way to the modern and immensely more efficient concept of taking the machine to the job.

Pallets

Although cases of heavy export cargo can be lifted as a single unit by inserting the forks of a truck between the battens, the pallet is the inseparable complement of the forklift truck. The earliest development, in 1947, from the primitive pallet included a metal ring at each corner. The "stevedore" pallet had arrived—a combination of the pallet and the landing board, familiar to many generations of dock workers. This was a functional change in pallet design. It was quickly followed by detailed changes which catered successfully for special types of cargo. For instance, that bogey of master stevedores, the bale of raw rubber—heavy, slippery, and very much alive—can now be imprisoned on a pallet provided with framework sides so that several highly individual bales become one cargo unit. Human ingenuity has succeeded in producing a pallet for every need. There is little excuse left for handling cargo as single packages.

Palletization

Seeing that there is an urgent need for creating the unit of cargo at the factory or as soon after as possible, it is worth remarking that very few port authorities have so far included palletization as a port service. At the Far Eastern port of Keelung, large tonnages of cement in paper bags are shipped. Left to itself this traffic would be a delaying element in the work of the port; the almost continuous rain to which Keelung is subject would make the handling of cement less than intermittent. When the bags are unloaded at the rear of the export shed they are placed on expendable pallets and the uniform load so obtained is strapped in position. Over this is placed a plastic cover that protects the bags from the rain. Taken to the ship's side by forklift truck, each pallet load is slung aboard and piled in the hold by a further forklift truck. The plastic envelope is returned to the shed for further use.

Even without the refinement of the protection against rain, a very real advantage has been gained by converting loose cargo into the unitized type. Pre-weighed pallets can reduce time taken in weighing loose cargo as well as reducing the actual handling. So long as export cargo is made up of homogeneous units—and in these days of cartons much of it is—the reduction in the number of handlings that immediately follows palletization should commend itself to shippers. The tangible appeal would doubtless come from reduced dock-handling charges and also lower rates at the destination port. Early palletization means that the advantage of larger units can be enjoyed from an earlier stage in the transportation process.

Pallet Pools

The simple objective of a pallet pool is to ensure that a user, wherever he may operate, has to his hand as many pallets as are needed and of the right type, in the right place at the right time. Considerable progress has been made in setting up pallet pools. Sweden, which country in 1949 settled on one standard size for its pallets, formed the first pool for Swedish Railways as far back as 1954. The European railway pool was largely based on Swedish experience. An interesting result of the widespread use of the standard pallet in that country has been to change the size of the lump of domestic sugar. This has been altered so that its new size creates consumer packages that fit consumer boxes and these in turn fit on to the pallet platform. The port of Manchester runs a successful pallet pool on very simple lines. A lorry driver who is delivering, say, a dozen pallet loads of export cargo on any of three standard-sized pallets, can pick up that number of similar sized empty pallets before leaving the dock. The documentation is of the simplest and the process saves time as against the normal breaking down of a fragmented load and the making up of pallet loads to be piled in the shed.

Port operators who have struggled with the many thousand cases of citrus fruit that make up a full cargo will appreciate the progress made at the port of Ashdod in Israel. In a recent season, 11 million half-boxes were palletized, with much saving in lorry times and in having more compact loads. Imported cargo is palletized in the ship's hold, and it remains in these pallets until broken down at the receivers' premises. This is possible because pallets form one large pool at the port from which exporters can draw as required.

The idea of expendable pallets where exporters and others faced the loss of the pallet after a single use has produced a variety of types in which the value of the pallet has been reduced. Now there is a very worth-while idea based on the discovery that many expendable pallets are still sound and capable of a second or third use where previously they have been discarded. Provided agreement could be reached on a few standard sizes, it is thought to be possible to operate a traffic by which usable TRANSIT pallets, as they will be marked, could be bought by local would-be users, at half the cost of a new pallet, from other users who have accumulated a stock of once-used TRANSITs. With the prospect of not having to scrap them, it is considered that exporters would be encouraged to have pallets of sounder material which would better stand the rigours of an intermodal journey.

In Great Britain a study conducted for the Ministry of Transport by a firm of American consultants has pronounced that a saving to industry of £4 million a year after 6 years and £18 million after 15 years could be made by instituting a national pallet pool, for which they make detailed proposals. There can be no doubt that the many transportation experts who hold out a brighter future for the pallet than for the container, base their conclusions largely on the operation ultimately of an international pallet pool. The early recognition (1958) by the British Customs of the pallet as a packing, freed it from import restrictions and made consideration of pallet pools possible. It has been estimated that the operation of a true pallet pool can increase savings by as much as 50 per cent even when those taking part in it are already committed to modern handling notions. The size of the problem is indicated by the fact that in 1965 there were more than 87 million wooden pallets produced and sold in the United States alone; this number is being added to each year.

Parallel with the development of the pallet and its extended use in ships' holds, forklift trucks have been produced particularly suited to working in confined spaces and these include the interior of a standard-sized container. There is a considerable future also for the pallet that operates on the principle of the air cushion for moving unitized cargo over horizontal distances. A 1-ton prototype of the air-cushion pallet was made in the autumn of 1966, and little imagination is required to predict how its successful development could revolutionize the movement of cargo—not only in dock sheds, warehouses, and the like places—but also in the 'tween decks of ships. Advantages are claimed to include the lightness of the equipment, its robustness, and its absence of component parts. Those that it does have are simple to replace. There is finger-tip control even of heavy loads which can easily be manœuvred into confined spaces. Minimum headroom is needed. There is no damage to floors by friction, and the loaded pallet can move over surfaces that would not be strong enough to support the weight of the accompanying forklift truck. The capital outlay and the running costs are low compared with other handling equipment; maintenance is said to be negligible. In the particularly demanding operations carried out in cold stores, this type of equipment is said to have a bright future.

The Conveyor

Prior to 1945 the conveyor had a very limited use in port operations. For the piling of bags, for the horizontal movement of bananas, meat, and a few other specialized traffics, conveyors had already proved their worth. Now they are used wherever homogeneous cargo has to be moved; many are built into the warehouse structure, working from floor to floor. Transportable conveyors have been found to be particularly useful for loading cartons, etc., into containers, especially the 40-foot type. Looking back over the decades, the most obvious feature of conveyor working would seem to have remained a secret; perhaps their potential value was not apparent until a comparison with cranes as an alternative lifting agent came to be made. Port operators had become so used to cranes that they had "thought" in terms of cranes and gantries. The hook had reigned supreme in dockland since the days of sail. It took a genius to point out what had always been obvious—that in the working cycle of a crane, or other equipment where there is dependence on a hook, less than 50 per cent of the time is spent on doing the job for which the crane was provided. Getting ready to lift the set, hooking it on, steadying the load for landing, unhooking the set, putting the used sling on to the hook and returning to the hold to commence the next cycle, all these operations leave only about 40 per cent of the time for the essential job of transferring the cargo from the hold to the quay. In so far as a crane is allowed to slew into a shed door, to ease the work of the quay gang, more time is wasted. This is a principle that has been accepted and applied in the working of the kangaroo-type of crane. Returning for another load is an inseparable part of crane working—the only exception that the ingenuity of man has so far devised is the container crane that takes a load in either direction (Fig. 20). The conveyor is the nearest approach to perpetual motion to be found in dockland. Long before 1939, experience had proved that the output of bananas, landed by pocket elevators on to horizontal conveyors, could easily beat the original method of landing the stems by packing them vertically into

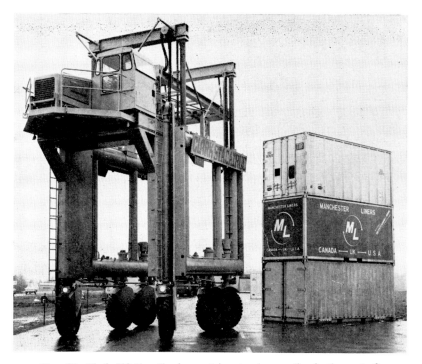

Fig. 20. Clark 512 Van Carrier container truck operating in the port of
Manchester. (By courtesy of Clark Stacatruc.)

large, padded trays from which they had each to be taken out on the
quays.

Minor Problems

In the early days of dock mechanization, so urgent was the need and so
compelling the volume of imports and exports to be handled, that there
was work for all dockers despite the reduced gangs that began to replace
the swollen hand gangs of 1939. However, as the work passed the empiric
stage and the pre-war piecework schedules became increasingly obsolete,
the problem of redundancy had to be faced. It has not yet been solved.

Certain precautions have had to be taken before it has been found
practicable to high-pile cargo. Not all carton cargo, for instance, will
stand up to the weight of 20 ft of similar cargo placed on top. Pallets have

been devised to take the stress on the four rigid corners rather than on the cargo itself, and this progress continues. Pallet racks are now a feature both in port and inland warehouses.

Many parties interested in the spread of mechanization have found it difficult to make the initial break-in. The process seems so complex that to alter any part would seem to invite the collapse of the conventional system without its being possible to replace it by a mechanized process. Where this is a real difficulty it can be overcome by a careful selection of the job to be treated. How to organize a container traffic for liners that load at a dozen different ports and discharge at ten, taking on more cargo during the voyage at intermittent ports, is a major problem not yet solved. To organize a simple shuttle service between two constant ports for a limited number of containers, very early proved to be a relatively simple matter. What cannot yet be done for the Far East traffic is simple for British Railways who carry containers regularly between Harwich and Zeebrugge. And yet this relatively minor achievement had to be worked out on lines that will one day solve the major problem. It was early learnt that the physical act of loading and discharging containers, the only part that the public saw, would always remain subservient to the more complex job of getting each cargo of containers to the loading port on time from all over the country and of disposing of them quickly at the port of discharge. In short, if you can select a simple form, preferably a shuttle service, on which to concentrate, success is more likely to come than by attacking a complicated structure. In attempting the latter, unlimited scope is provided for those who, by nature and training, see in every solution one more difficulty.

In the past the standard of marking cargo, the means by which the docker separates the contents of each bill of lading, left much to be desired. Bad and insufficient marking, to which reference has already been made, has long been recognized as one of the major hidden difficulties in achieving better ship turnround. It was the first major study commenced in 1957 by the recently formed International Cargo Handling Co-ordination Association. The findings published by that body on the marking of general cargo are still applicable, and have been accepted internationally. They have also been widely publicized by cargo-loss prevention committees and underwriters. Under the urge for mechanization there has been real progress in the standard of cargo marking. Simple codes on green fruit have replaced a multitude of growers' private marks. Small bills of lading and bad, insufficient, or unnecessarily complicated systems of marking have been recognized as the enemies of mechanization. They are losing the battle because anything that handicaps the docker must be tackled, whatever private interests of long standing are concerned.

The Three Laws of Mechanization

When the pioneers of mechanization found time to detach their thoughts from the next day's approaching crisis—and all dock work has been defined as moving quietly from one crisis to the next—they realized that they had stumbled on a new science and not something that could be dismissed as a series of very interesting but unrelated experiments. Perhaps the first major discovery that emerged, and the re-thinking was taking place independently at all the major ports, was a recognition of the functional nature of each machine. To confine it to its proper function was an essential step forward. With this as a firm basis from which to advance, three principles (or laws as they came to be recognized) were gradually evolved.

The first law was dimly realized; it had been applied long before 1939. The major scientific intervention into port work during the inter-war years was the electric truck. Used in the early 1920s to speed up the disposal of the cargo from the ship's side and to cut down the damage that was part of hand-truck work, it was soon borne in on the port officer that speed in removing cargo called for a similar speeding up, both in the ship's hold and in the rail and road vehicles into which the cargo was to be loaded. With immediate-delivery cargo, taken away by rail wagons, the hourly shunt that took out full wagons and replaced them with empties, now had to be done every 20 minutes. This affected the railway company's organization right back to the marshalling yard. Owners of lorries found that loading time was drastically cut; more lorries had to be put on the run so as to keep the ship working at the higher rate made possible by the abolition of hand trucking. Perishable cargo, such as meat and fruit, now arrived earlier at the central markets.

Put into words the first law ran: "If you improve a stage in the process of cargo handling you will immediately have to improve the stage before and immediately after that one."

The second law emerged when the port operator found time to ask himself a very pertinent question. The answer to this question had, and will have for many years, shattering results. WHAT DO WE DO IN THE DOCKS?

The answer is simple—we pick things up and we put them down again in another place; sometimes in another form. When the units of cargo are in excess of the number that can be picked up and put down by the available labour, in the time that it is willing to work, then congestion will arise with its attendant evils. Port work having been reduced to its simplest definition, the obvious step was to produce the larger unit of cargo, so that each picking up and putting down again would—with no increase in mechanical effort—speed the flow of cargoes across the quays.

From the acceptance of this idea came the unit-load and palletized cargo, also the revolutionary conception, to the timber trade, of packaged timber; eventually the optimum of the general-cargo world—the container. Practical difficulties prevented many of the earlier unit loads from having any but a short life. Dislike of pallets in the ship's hold and the need to use forklift trucks for wing stowage meant that, while export cargo could be palletized on arrival at the rear of the export shed, these pallet loads were broken down in the ship's hold. Each part of the unit load was then stowed as an individual package.

The second law can be put into words: "The unit of cargo should be the largest that is practicable; it must remain as a unit for the longest possible time in its journey from producer to consumer."

The third law followed very quickly from the acceptance of the long-life principle of the unit load. To get the biggest saving from these loads, mechanical handling must be exploited to the full. Individually the unit load must be as large or as heavy as the available machine can handle. Anything less than this amounts to under-use; this can be seen every day when the set of madeup packages, seldom weighing more than 25 cwt, is lifted by the 3- or 5-ton crane. To exploit this expensive machinery it must be used either as single items of equipment or as a combination of facilities for the maximum number of working hours. In other words, all cargo must be so prepared as to permit of mechanical handling; cargo handled manually must become a dwindling exception. Producers of cargo-handling equipment must study the conditions of port-work and accept the fact that these make demands on them far more exacting than the factory or the depot. The general-purpose machine is more to be desired than the specialized unit packed away in vaseline for half the year. Mechanical handling for the largest possible tonnage of cargo passing through a port demands many types of machines before the third law can be applied. This is a corollary to the second law and it runs: "The process of mechanization must be commenced at the earliest possible stage in the journey from producer to consumer and it must be maintained for the longest practical portion of the journey."

Handling costs will, therefore, be in inverse proportion to the amount of mechanization that the nature of the cargo permits and the ingenuity of the port operator can devise.

If a fourth law can be invisaged as emerging from the discovery and application of the three described above, it would be worded somewhat on these lines: "The cost of living in a maritime country will be influenced largely by the success with which the three laws that govern the mechanical handling of cargo can be applied."

The Mechanical Equipment Committee

Reverting to the initial difficulties of introducing mechanization, particularly in ports where there is rooted objection to any reduction in labour or where physical conditions are not favourable, it is important to grasp that the revolution can never be brought about by one man. To be successful it must be the co-ordinated effort helped forward by the port operator, the engineer, and the purchasing officer. Together they should form a committee known for convenience as the Mechanical Equipment Committee. To make its finding effective it is advisable that each operating member should have the responsibility of carrying out the decisions of the committee in his part of the port. What is the work to be done by a Mechanical Equipment Committee? The first job is to consider the functions of mechanical equipment and assess the ways in which the separate items can be employed to speed the work of the port; from this survey it is possible to determine the most serviceable types of equipment that should be purchased having regard to the problems and the working conditions set by the cargo handled. Continual study of the extended use of equipment will be necessary so as to avoid multiplying the types, with the consequent need to carry large stocks of spares. All the time the eyes of the committee must be fixed on acquiring general purpose rather than specialized machines. Particular care must be paid to formulating a maintenance programme which will be run in conjunction with a "withdrawal from use" programme rigidly enforced. The committee will be required to study carefully the working conditions, to analyse accidents to determine their causes (and there will be many accidents during the early stages), and to produce rules for safe working of the machines and

T.F.P.—D

the safety of their drivers. The proper observance of standing orders will introduce uniformity in working and make for a simple interchange of machines and drivers. The training of the latter is an important part of the committee's work. Drivers will not be allowed to take machines into dock use until they (the drivers) have passed a test set by the dock engineer; each qualified driver will be given a certificate of proficiency and this will be withdrawn if a high standard of performance is not maintained. As well as the above the committee will keep an eye on physical conditions, particularly as the process is extended. Quays, sheds, and gangways may need a radical overhaul before they become capable of getting the best out of the new and expensive equipment.

As experience is gained the committee may find it necessary from time to time to co-opt a principal officer of the port authority to advise on a certain aspect of mechanization. A secretary, not being a member of the committee, will call meetings which should be at regular intervals, keep the minutes, and record the decisions of the committee. Minutes should be numbered consecutively from the first meeting and couched in a form that can be used as operating orders for the staff. Further, it may be found advisable in ports where there is a training school for drivers to have the principal of this as a permanent member of the committee. The intervals between meetings should not be so short as to prevent enough material to be gathered for a full agenda, nor so long that items become outdated. A meeting every 2 weeks has been found a practical way of keeping the subject in the foreground. If meetings can take place at the same time of day and in the same place, the Mechanical Equipment Committee will become a live feature in the working life of the port and also of each of its members.

CHAPTER 6

LABOUR I

Introduction

The earlier chapters of this book have described the modern port, the ships, the berths, and the cargoes that are handled there. They are handled by port labour—by stevedores who load and discharge the cargo, and the dock workers who, in addition sometimes to performing the ship discharge, are responsible for the picking up and putting down again of millions of cargo units on the quays and in the sheds and warehouses.[1] Inseparable from the men handling cargo is the force of lightermen who manœuvre the craft that provide so valuable an outlet for the overside loading or discharge of general goods. Only rarely, in such ports as Manchester in England, where conditions do not allow of barge working, can the lightermen be left out of the picture. Complementary also are the dock railway workers who operate the internal rail system. Not to be ignored is the large force of lorry drivers employed in a multitude of trades but all having a common interest in an efficiently run port and themselves contributing directly to this end.

No study of port labour would be of value without recognizing the changes that have taken place since 1945 in the nature of the cargo handled, the equipment now available for handling it, and the demands made on port workers under modern conditions. It would have been tedious to have constantly drawn attention to the contribution which each invention in the design of ships, each new approach to unitizing cargo, and the almost daily improvement in handling equipment has made in reducing the demand for the services of port workers. To appreciate how every recent trend in port work has spelt out the same answer—fewer men needed —it is necessary to recall the busy scenes prior to 1939 when a far greater

---

[1] Disputes involving the staffing of container depots away from the docks point to the need for a new definition of dock work. A sub-committee to define "the vicinity of the port" was appointed (November 1969) in Great Britain.

number of packages than are at present handled had to be picked up, moved, and put down again singly and in small units, very largely by hand truckmen.

Port Work—The Nature of

Many port operators can still recall the conditions of those inter-war years. Port work had reached a static stage and output and ship turnround was broadly satisfactory to the shipping companies. Conditions of work, although still largely on a casual basis, compared favourably with those in other industries. Despite some changes for the better that the last two decades have seen, the industry still contains many points that are unsatisfactory to the employers and inherently unattractive to labour. This static background is made up of some features that neither legislation nor changing cargo conditions can ever entirely alter.

Firstly, there is the casual nature of all port work. In the 1820s, when the first attempt was made to schedule liner sailings and men pretended to see, with the growing use of steam, an end to the casual comings and goings of cargo vessels, the weather factor refused to be ignored. Neither can it be entirely ignored 150 years later. Seasonal changes can to an extent be predicted; political changes can, without notice, close a few miles of water connecting the Mediterranean Sea and the Indian Ocean, causing shipping to be diverted and depriving port labour for weeks of their expected work. This has happened twice in recent years. Budget changes following on devaluation cause a search for alternative sources of supply. Similarly, tariff changes abroad make possible an increase in certain exports. Industrial troubles in one country will cause cargoes to be diverted to another country and, as labour is in process of learning, nothing is easier to re-route than a ship full of cargo. A major port may note that the demand for labour within its docks varies on two successive days by 9000 men; this does not make news. If it is not possible to predict with any certainty the daily demand for labour, how can port employers form an estimate for a few years ahead?

Dock work is becoming increasingly specialized. The Victorian docker with pride in his muscle and endurance and with ample opportunity to exercise both, is out of date. The skill of the stevedore with his hook, his mastery of the heavy cargo that he manipulated, and his use of gravity made him irreplaceable. Putting a hand to a container, driving a container crane or a forklift truck—all these could be done by women—a fact that few dockers care to face. No physical effort is now needed to achieve phenomenal gang-hour tonnages.

History of Port Labour

A handicap under which both sides work in a port is the unhappy history of port labour. Looking briefly at the enclosed ports of the United Kingdom we can trace a sincere effort in their formative days for the work to be done by labour hired on permanent conditions. With the haphazard handling of a multitude of small cargo ships, berthed in tiers in tidal conditions in the River Thames, labour was casually employed. Not one of the many hundred employers would accept responsibility for the welfare of the "mudlarks", as the eighteenth century ship labour in London was then called. With the arrival of the dock companies there was a general move towards elevating the status of their labour. An establishment, fixed at several hundred men for each of the new docks, very quickly came up against the facts of life, even in the new phase that the docks presented. Although this revolutionized port working it could not alter the weather. An adverse wind that held for some weeks at a time, cluttered the estuarial waters with sail by the hundred. The new docks, only a few score miles away, remained empty, the demand for labour fell, and the dock companies had their shareholders to think about. Not even an organization of philanthropists could maintain a fixed establishment that was seldom in touch with the realities of the work. It was recognized by both sides that the supply of labour must be flexible. In the thinking of the period, and in fact until 1967, the only practical way of achieving this was by casual labour. The establishment of the dock companies became the sport of economics. Each was increased as the company foresaw, or thought that it did, a semi-permanent improvement in the volume of work. Nothing was simpler than to reduce the establishment when this predicted improvement failed to last. Regretfully the dock company became resigned to a pattern that they saw unfolding and which still rules today—an alternation of booms and slumps. Casual labour was the only expedient that could cope with such conditions.

In their need to economize—and not many dock companies were ever prosperous—the proprietors turned their attention to the overall costs that every employer faces in the act of paying the men he employs. During most of the nineteenth century, dock work was simple enough to be put out to contractors, and this was done through the dock superintendent.

As was to be expected in the conditions that ruled, contractors cut each others' throats to secure the work; the arrangements they made to pay the men they employed were subject to no national nor even port agreement. Everything depended on the overriding conditions of supply and demand. When work was scarce the rate for the job fell. Conversely, during the 1880s, when the country enjoyed a period of prosperity, the contractor was forced to pay more to secure his share of dependable labour. Whatever troubles the contractor ran into, the dock company paid him a flat rate per ton. Administrative costs on both sides remained minimal.[1] Social historians of the period comment severely on the degradation brought on labour by this system of contract working; the last of the contractors faded from the Surrey Commercial Docks in London in 1924.

The Piecework System

Several decades before Henry Ford discovered that the best employer is the one that contrives—and "contrives" is the operative word—to pay the highest rate for the job, the dock companies began to flirt with the idea of piecework. Some of the more intelligent labourers saw in a system, operated by the proprietors, a relief from the selfishly inhuman conditions imposed by the contractors, where a man was "too old at forty". They also saw a chance to improve their earnings above the daywork payments which were all that they could expect however long they remained in the industry. The companies hesitated long before they sanctioned a system that was administratively expensive and out of which they had no guarantee that working costs per ton would fall. However, by the 1880s some operations were being done on direct piecework, and it was a condition of the settlement of the Great Strike in London of 1889 that advances should be energetically made on the number of operations done on piecework. To the layman it seemed that nothing but good could come out to both sides from converting dock work entirely to piecework. The docker could exert himself knowing that his effort would be rewarded. The employer would know the basic cost of every operation with the certainty that his overhead costs would fall as his tonnage rose. All that remained was for both sides to agree, firstly, on the tonnage that, for each operation, would represent a fair day's work. Secondly, on the rate to be paid for every ton

---

[1] The contractor's paper-work, such as it was, was usually done in a local pub. The practice by master stevedores of paying their men "on the case" at the close of work persisted in London until the late 1920s.

handled. In practice, labour held back until a rate was agreed. Then it went all out to earn big money only to have the employer cut back the rate. This process of "pull devil, pull baker" came into the docks with piecework; it has been going on ever since. The system also presupposed perfect, or at least normal, working conditions. Unfortunately, conditions in dock work are not always normal; cargo becomes damaged in transit, it can be stowed in an awkward way in the hold, cargo-handling gear can be ineffective or not available. In a dozen ways the ingenuity of the worker can claim an allowance for the unfavourable conditions the job presents and the reduced output that not even an extra effort will avoid. Human nature being what it is, it is natural that the daily interpretation of piecework rates provides a breeding ground for disputes, arguments, and only too often stoppages that are not confined to the job in hand. Demands are pitched absurdly high in the certain knowledge that they will be cut; it has come to be considered legitimate to take every advantage of the ship's need to sail or of her scheduled engagements in her next port of call. To finish a cotchel of cargo to enable a ship to catch a tide, an unreasonable working of overtime or the fabrication of a demand made by misrepresenting conditions that are perfectly normal, has developed a new principle of working—the "either–else" method. In operating this, labour holds most of the cards. The stakes from the shipping company's angle are too high for them to fight back; to give way is simple and the ship sails.

In this unhealthy atmosphere, where no statement could be taken at its face value and where labour's signature to an agreement came to be valueless, many thinking men saw the only solution in a radical alteration of the basic conditions of employment. It was true that "work or reasonable support", the corner stone of the National Dock Labour Board schemes, had not only operated since 1941 in British ports, but had been copied in several foreign ports. Time had revealed the imperfections of a plan conceived under the administratively simple conditions of the Second World War. Under the scheme labour mobility was curtailed and many hours were wasted in sending surplus labour to places where it could be employed. It was common knowledge that employers hoarded labour against the overnight arrival of their next ship rather than return men to the pool. Conversely, having a certain knowledge of the kind of labour likely to be available next day, employers cut down on their demands, dockers were then thrown back into the pool, and vessels were undermanned until such time as a reluctant employer had to part with "choice" gangs. Once more human nature did its best to wreck a scheme which started by promising both sides a fair deal only to discover that neither side wanted one; both sides schemed to avoid having one imposed on them.

The scheme did nothing to "institutionalise" dock labour. It was possible for a pool labourer to work for eleven employers during the eleven working periods of the then working week. Few pool men were able to secure a lien on the work of one of the larger employers. Few pool men belonged or felt that they belonged to an employer. While these drawbacks, and others, were known to exist, while restrictive practices by labour were matched by irresponsible practices by the employers, neither side had confidence that they could, either separately or in co-operation, devise a better system. Both sides would have agreed to its abolition if a better one could, overnight, have been put in its place.

On 18 September 1967 port labour became decasualized in all the ports of Great Britain. Before looking at some of the effects of this most momentous of all steps in the long and unhappy history of port labour, it will be necessary to look first at some of the practical conditions in which the daily work of the docks is done.

Making dock workers permanent has left many of these unchanged.[1]

How Conditions Work Against High Output

In industry sound management and foresighted planning have a reasonable chance of ensuring a profitable output. In port work it would seem that every aspect has been put there in order to frustrate the effort of the employer. Unlike the factory, where the workers move every day on to machines made familiar by use, and the safety of whose working is assured, a dock is full of ships that do not belong to the port authority nor, very likely, to the master stevedore whose labour works the holds. The nature of the cargo, the amount of work to be done, and the processes which may have to be employed, vary from day to day or even from hour to hour, and may not always be known in advance. Neither is the gear, be it quay crane or ship's winch, certain to be the property of the port employer. The operators may have neither pride in its operation nor assurance of its stability. That this doubt is a real one was demonstrated recently in a

[1] Since decasualization costs have risen 30 per cent and productivity has fallen about 30 per cent—a statement made in July 1969 by the chairman of the London Port Employers.

United Kingdom port by the refusal of a master stevedore to handle cargo stowed in pre-slung sets. He would, he urged, be held responsible for an accident to one of his men should a sling, the property of the master stevedore at the loading port, prove defective.

The fact that even under decasualization men can be "lent" between employers shows how unpracticable it has proved to be in abolishing the casual nature of the work. The move to decasualize port labour followed some research into the number of men that each employer could take and the average age of dockworkers; it is confirmation of the arduous conditions of the work and the unattractive surroundings in which much of it is performed that it has in an age of full employment failed to recruit the younger and more active workers. It is true that with the shadow of decasualization hanging over the industry, recruitment of pool workers was stopped 6 years ago in the United Kingdom ports. It is also a fact that the mass of dockers are over 40—the biggest single age group in the industry is that between 55 and 59; in other words, a large proportion of the 55,000 pool workers in the country were pre-1939 entrants to the industry. For an industry to contain so many men in the upper age groups is not a healthy feature.

Weather conditions are generally adverse (Fig. 21). A ship's hold can be unpleasantly hot in summer; a quay shed is certainly unpleasantly cold in winter. The Far East port of Keelung has more than 200 days of rain each year. It is not generally practicable to give protection against this, and local labour has come to ignore it.

If there were a constant desire on both sides to reach an amicable settlement to every dispute—one does not use the word "fair" because in port work it has ceased to have meaning—the many stoppages, minor strikes, overtime bans, and the like that dog the employers' efforts to turn ships round, would not be so deplorable a feature of the industry. Always there is the fear of redundancy; more will be said of this shadow that has darkened the labour horizon since the first forklift truck was left behind by a returning United States port unit in 1945 at Tilbury Dock. Shift work, seen by the dockers as a threat, can be used as a bargaining counter in productivity agreements; the withdrawal of overtime working has generally reduced normal work in major ports to an 8-hour day. Although no new feature, the unofficial leader has caught the imagination of the public and the front page of the Press. In no other industry could a very ordinary union member bring out not only the port workers of his own

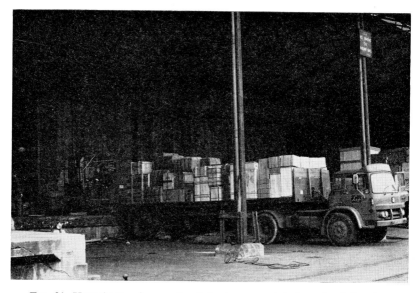

FIG. 21. How the London weather is beaten; exports being unloaded under the protection of a canopy built at the end of an export shed.
(By courtesy of PLA.)

port but inflict an unofficial national dock strike which, for several weeks, the unions failed to settle.[1]

Since the General Strike of 1926 all efforts in the United Kingdom to combine port workers into one union have failed. The "Blue" Union—a few thousand very militant and well disciplined stevedores—have been at enmity with the mammoth "White" union. For 40 years they have continued to fight each other, rarely putting up a joint front against the employer, who has seen his best schemes constantly bedevilled by this interunion dissension. With blue labour on the ship and, owing to the crazy pattern of port labour in London, white labour often on the quay, there has been ample room for irritation. This has often been caused by the

[1] This is because an individual can be the spark to the gunpowder and the gunpowder is provided by the circumstances which consist of the historical background of the industry, including the attitude of employers within the industry in other days. This is the considered view of a union leader who discounts the theory of the dynamic personality of the unofficial leader.

outdated system of conciliation where members of both unions are concerned. Similarly, when new port ventures are conceived, trouble is almost certain as the blue union see the likelihood of their members not receiving what they consider to be a proper share of the work. However, the major problems that followed on decasualization have introduced a more sensible approach and, at last, a joint working and advisory committee of the two unions has been set up. If it works, and there is no reason against this, one of the major self-imposed handicaps under which port labour has for a lifetime worked, should disappear.

Although decasualization should have meant less power to promote stoppages, the Continuity Rule, a strictly Second World War measure, has now the sacred-cow status of a port custom. In 1943 ships with unpopular cargoes were boycotted by labour and remained in port for a long time. It was enacted, as a war measure only, that men sent by the Dock Board should remain at work on the hold allocated until it was finally discharged. It is still in operation and has, since 1946, been a frequent cause of stoppages and disputes.

Working Conditions

Although, broadly speaking, dock work is regulated by national agreements, there are differences in the local interpretation of agreements. Neither is there international agreement on hours, payments, or systems of working. In some countries these are influenced by a permanent shortage of labour that has, in the Netherlands, been met by imported labour. In North Africa employment is spread over a permanent surplus of labour so that every man may have a similar allocation of port work. However, there are some principles that it has been found, in the interests of higher output, advantageous to apply. In the present state of port labour piecework is still in many ports the main condition before tonnage can be secured. There are healthy signs that we may be moving out of this phase, now some 80 years old; these will be described later. A form of piecework can certainly be applied even when conditions are basically unsuitable, as with the "Group" system built up on patriarchal lines in some Far East ports.

It is accepted generally by both sides that the gang should be made up of essential men only. A gang discharging loose general cargo ashore should be composed of the hatchwayman (the ganger), two winchdrivers, and three pairs working down below making the cargo into sets for landing.

In this tight little organization each man is essential to the task the gang has been set; the work of each is balanced so that each man is permanently employed while not being overstrained. In practice the hatchwayman can supervise the making up of the sets and can guide each one safely ashore. The two winchdrivers work continuously and in harmony to transfer the sets ashore, and the three pairs down below in rotation and at a speed that allows each pair "to sit on their sets" for a spell of a few minutes. If there were only two pairs they would be worked to a standstill; if there were six, half of the men would be "waiting for the hook". The output of the whole gang is such as to keep the winches or the crane working an uninterrupted cycle. This produces cargo for the receiving gang on the quay to handle at the maximum pace for which this gang has been constructed. When it is found possible to increase output per crane or winch cycle, either by making up larger sets or reducing the time of the cycle, then the size of the gang on the ship, and in turn the gang on the quay, can be adjusted to conform. Similarly, if cargo has been damaged and is difficult to get out, a reduced gang only on the quay is necessary. If export cargo has to be lifted from the quay and each set lowered to the ceiling of a large passenger ship, the crane cycle will be so extended as to limit the number of men needed both in the hold and in serving the ship.

Success of piecework depends on several factors. The most important is that every man in the gang should know what his job is, how it fits in with that done by every other man in the gang, and—most essential— that he should be able to see that each man is making his due contribution to the gang's output. The target tonnage must have been agreed beforehand; it should be a reasonable target that can be achieved without strain. There must be no interference with the rhythm of the job through documentary or administrative delays. Well-organized piecework will also help to ensure a good standard of timekeeping.[1]

Reasonable discipline will be ensured by simple and effective supervision exercised by foremen shipworkers and foremen quay-gangers promoted from the ranks of labour. The extent of the piecework bill must be controlled; the ideal bill should not run for more than two consecutive shifts. Thus if through weather or other drawbacks conditions do not promote high earnings, the bill can be shut down and the loss written off. To do

---

[1] Where teamwork has replaced piecework it has, on one berth in London, been found practicable to induce men to report a quarter of an hour before the official starting time to collect clothing and gear.

this is more conducive to high output than saddling the bill with a deficit that the men know they cannot wipe out during the tenure of the bill.

From 1957 to 1959 the Pacific Maritime Association and the International Longshoremens' and Warehousemens' Union worked out the details of an agreement which enabled the employers to introduce mechanical cargo-handling methods with liberalized working rules. The men of the registered working force were to be protected from loss of work and to a share in the savings made possible by mechanization. The agreement which came into force in 1960 included a guaranteed wage of $116 for a 35-hour working week. The union agreed that men could be switched during shift (either singly or in gangs) from ship to pier, from ship to ship, or from pier to pier to reduce labour "dead time". The employers also agreed to pay *to the union* $5 million a year—to a maximum of $29·5 million during the term of the agreement—to enable the union to "buy out" redundant workers by means of full pensions and early retirement payments. The maximum payment to any single worker was $7920. The agreement was re-negotiated for a further period in 1966. Mr. Paul St. Sure, president of the employers' association, stated that "the agreement provides a blueprint for employers to operate as an efficient management and take advantage of the agreement without taking advantage of the men". Mr. H. Bridges, president of the union, said: "Anyone who knows anything about the industry knows that 'gold is only found' when ships get a fast turnround. This is the root and base of the agreement. We are determined to make it work because the basic principles it sets forth are sound and good for the men."

The San Francisco Port Study, carried out in 1958–9, showed that delays accounted for about 43 per cent of the working time in the holds. That unproductive time at the beginning and end of shifts accounted for a further 7 per cent and that inflexible gang sizes prevented the efficient utilization of manpower. It was this kind of situation that the agreement was designed to correct. Its re-negotiation after $5\frac{1}{2}$ years testing period suggests that, with good will and common sense on both sides, solutions can be found.

Each man must know the amount of his "take home" pay. This should be an exact fraction of the bill's earning according to the number of men in the gang. No bill should be allowed to carry "passengers" nor should deductions for unofficial payments be tolerated. Payments should be made to labour at recognized and regular times. Whilst these conditions would seem elementary to an efficient port operator, failure to ensure that they are normal port practice is a certain way of losing output. Frequent and excessive overtime, although favoured by many dock workers as a certain means of swelling their pay packet, should be avoided. The working alternative is a two-shift system, and the effort needed to get this adopted is worthwhile in view of the flexibility this provides. Objections, mainly on account of the disruption of domestic life, are many; agreement on the hours to be worked, both in length and the time of day, will call for some re-thinking.[1] There is real need to move away from the rigid 8-hour 8–5 strait-jacket that has ruled United Kingdom ports since the Shaw Award of 1920 and has made the foreigner marvel that United Kingdom ports are unworked for two-thirds of their time.[2] Particularly for specialized berth working, such as the new grain terminal at Tilbury Dock in London, is the agreement to speed ship turnround by shift working to be welcomed.

There are many who claim that given a sufficiency of regular and efficient sea services, with the right equipment to handle them, the piecework system will provide a consistently higher output than daywork. Unfortunately, as in so many port controversies, it is seldom, if ever, possible to compare like with like. Since piecework began to predominate as the desire for an incentive grew, it came to be accepted that effort should produce around 30 per cent payment additional to the day rates; this, later, was guaranteed and it led to a complete loss of interest in the bad jobs, the deficit on which the management had to pay. There is so much difference between the berth, the ship, and the general conditions of cargo, that little can be done in the attempt by both sides to have cover for every calculable condition. The piecework schedule has become a huge and unwieldy tome. Out of this the unofficial leader can dig an argument in favour of higher pay. If, for instance, a cargo of fertilizer received in bad condition is rewarded with an extra shilling (5p) a ton for discharging, then it is all too easy for labour to maintain that the next cargo is equally damaged. The tendency for the exceptional to become the normal is difficult to resist. In the early days of the system, when management and the unions had adequate control of the men and when agreements made

---

[1] It will certainly need adjustment in the transport system serving the port.
[2] One container berth at Tilbury Dock in London is now worked from 7 a.m. until midnight. Ship working finishes usually at 7 p.m., but receiving and delivering cargo goes on till midnight. The second shift is based on a rota system; late workers are free on the following day.

were automatically honoured, it worked well. Now it is ammunition placed ready to the hand of the trouble maker.

Manning for Mechanized Piecework

In many industries manning for mechanized gangs provides problems the solutions for which are not acceptable to labour. There are certainly many problems in port work that, even given 100 per cent co-operation by both sides, would from a practical angle still seem to be insoluble. Where the process is repetitive, where it is in the order of things that the machine used, the material handled, and the type of labour are unalterable, when it is known, further, that this will always be the case, goodwill on both sides can hammer out a solution. The major problem with ship's cargoes, however, is how to mechanize the work rather than how to man the job. Whilst cargoes of bulk grain, bananas, meat, and timber provide a certainty that work of the same character will persist throughout the process of discharge, general cargo consists of a variety of packages of differing size, shape, and weight. Not all are capable of being handled alongside other cargo. The design of the ship, the port premises, the barge, and how the cargo is stowed in the ship and how it is to be stowed in the shed or the barge, determine the size of the gang that can be employed. Whereas export cargo can be, and generally is, palletized on arrival at the docks and remains in this form until the unit is broken down in the ship's hold, it is not always practicable (although progress in this direction has been made) for pallets to be used as landing boards for bringing import cargo ashore. Moreover, this method of handling exports does not comply, as we have shown in the previous chapter, with the fundamental laws of mechanization. The cargo stowed in general-cargo ships is usually mixed; bills of lading have to be worked out in their entirety because they are needed ashore, or in the barge, intact. It is rarely possible to work across a hold and down at the same time. Sorting is an essential part of discharge; the greater the number of bills of lading carried by the ship the more sorting is necessary.

When a day's work from one hold may include unmixed loose goods, casks, heavy cases, loose timber, bales of rubber, and crates of hardboard, each of which calls for a different-sized gang, then, if the benefits of mechanization are to be enjoyed by the employer, the problem he faces is obvious. The commodities mentioned, if there were enough of them to provide 8 hours' uninterrupted work, could be handled on the ship economically and mechanically by gangs varying in size from three to sixteen men. Similarly, gangs to receive such cargo would vary as the day wore on. Years of experience have shown that a composite gang of an agreed size will be able to handle nearly all types of loose cargo. Certain cargoes will require less or more men for which provision can be, and is, made. No berth can be worked satisfactorily when four or five times a day the composition of the gang, and also the equipment used, has to be replaced because the cargo for which it has been designed has given out.

Some years ago a shipping line brought cargo consisting of mixed Scandinavian wood and wood goods to London. These were tediously sorted on board to bill of lading quantity, each being delivered to a separate barge at a necessarily deliberate pace. In conjunction with the Port of London Authority the method was replaced by a total landing of all the cargo; this was made up on pallets immediately prior to landing. They were received on the quay by forklift trucks, run into the shed, and piled to bills of lading; provision for this had been made by bedding out the shed beforehand. Overside deliveries from water-served berths were made at the rear of the shed; this was done in conjunction with road deliveries. Two ships on this run were soon doing the work previously done by three, and a further berth was converted to this method. This case illustrates a fundamental difficulty and one method by which it has been solved. To have cargo already in unit form or to have it in a form that permits of quick and safe unitization is the only way by which a mechanized manning scale can be applied. As we have said earlier, the simpler the pilot experiment, the more likely it is that the ultimate transfer to the new method will be successful. The very gradual process of unitizing the products of the factory at, or before the factory door, is making steady progress—there are so many arguments in its favour. Only after its transfer from the package to the unit can mechanization begin. Some employers have dodged the question by supplying mechanical equipment while leaving the gang the same size as for manual operations. They hope that when the men learn to handle the new equipment it may be possible to reduce their number.

Package Deals

Nothing remains unchanged for many decades in the port industry. Because cargoes and conditions are constantly altering, labour requirements also call for change. We have seen how piecework replaced daywork.

Coming in as a more equitable alternative to the contractor and his discredited methods, it soon became clear that certain rigid conditions were necessary before piecework could be operated in a manner acceptable to the men. Gangs of agreed size must be present at the start of the job, machinery must be in good condition, and the cargo, if it was not in perfect shape on arrival, would attract an allowance by way of compensation. Very quickly dockers became perfectionists. A rigidity not hitherto known when men received a fixed sum at the end of a day's work, crept in. Not only had the cargo to be in good condition and well stowed; a lighterman must be present to receive goods before they were put into his craft by the ship's gang. It is now many years since a lighterman has put a hand to the cargo that, before piecework, he took an active part in stowing. The work would not start without a tally clerk, ready with his card and pencil to record an out-turn that could be—and has been done in an emergency—by the winchdriver on his winch-end. After the Second World War, gangs would not start if they were one or more men short; neither would the unions permit the obvious remedy of "milking" one gang to make up the others. One could daily encounter the crazy conditions where all six gangs placed on a general cargo-ship at 8 a.m. were each one man short. Six incomplete gangs sat on the deck and did nothing until they could be made up at 1 p.m. call. In many similar ways the work was delayed—"piecework will keep, what's the hurry". The contention that the dockers do not come to the dock to work but to impose their own interpretation of a national agreement—the Rule Book as it is called—what time they are not holding a pistol at the head of the employer by manipulating piecework conditions, gained increasing credibility among the long-suffering employers.

And then in 1947 the first roll-on roll-off service, run with wartime LSTs, commenced to operate from London. As well as vehicles, a few tons of mails were carried, shipped over the quay. Parcels of general cargo were accepted, for a speedy delivery to the Continent was guaranteed. The proprietors realized that to conform in all ways to the piecework schedule or to attempt to pay a tonnage rate on vehicles, to the shipment of which the dockers had made no physical contribution, would be a certain road to bankruptcy, albeit preserving the sacred cow of the Rule Book. Selecting a small gang with some care, the company fixed a weekly wage in excess of that paid for normal package traffic, and for the first time the dockers got on with the work irrespective of conditions that ruled, whether cargo was being loaded or discharged, or both at the same time. Naturally the men concerned were satisfied with a deal that was the envy of the rest of the dock and a direct flouting of the all-powerful unions. It has worked for many years; it was the prototype agreement for a system that is making progress by putting the clock back. To drag dock work into the second half of the twentieth century it is necessary to go back 100 years.

New berths built for container and unit-load traffic have produced working conditions to meet which the conventional piecework schedule is as suitable as the penny-farthing bicycle on a motorway. By August 1967 there were four berths in the port of London where a guaranteed wage had replaced earnings by piecework.[1] More important was the acceptance by the men concerned of the principle that they were there to do work waiting to be done, but this came as a later development. Opposition by one union was based on the argument that phase 2 of the Devlin plan for modernization was being rushed and that so great a disregard of the Rule Book should not be made without some bargaining arising from decasualization. The other union thought that it would penalize those groups of men who would never catch up, for a package deal would attract the more active and go-ahead workers prepared to disregard the book for the bigger wage packet. The first master stevedore to formulate a package offer was inundated with applicants. Both sides, and this the unions conceded, were certain that by removing the catch-as-catch-can atmosphere, into which the piecework system had deteriorated, a better understanding between employer and docker would quickly emerge. The berths first selected for the experiment catered for special traffics, but the record outputs achieved and maintained from the start owed much to the new enthusiasm brought to the job by men working as a team and not as a gang. In the case of a new venture in timber and timber products, some of the dockers were sent to the Swedish terminal of the company to see for themselves how the cargo could be handled. Packaged timber has proved an ideal traffic for team work, and at the new berths in the Port of London outputs that were at first regarded as phenomenal are now normal. It has been described by the leading employer as "good for the men, good for the shippers, and good for the port". Bulk grain is now being handled by a team of specialized labour, traditionally conventional in their outlook

---

[1] The stability and security of a realistic weekly wage is attractive after the fluctuations and uncertainties of the piecework system of payment.

and known as "cornporters". Overtime and other problems enabling work to be started irrespective of the time of arrival of the ship on the berth, have been settled amicably, bringing a new spirit into some parts of dockland.

The major breakthrough has been made at a general-cargo berth in London where the more forward-looking dockers, regarding the traffic lost recently to other ports, have formed themselves into a team pledged, literally, to come to the dock to get the job done despite the many obstacles that are inherent in the industry. Only by taking this line, they realize, can conditions be made attractive to shipowners. In this day and age new traffic is constantly looking for a suitable berth; this they interpret as part of the dock where the workpeople will go out of their way to help and to assist shipowners who have difficult cargoes to discharge, are pressed for time, and in fact look to labour for the help that many years ago a shipowner thought he had the right to expect. That this policy is already paying dividends is proved by the increase of work already booked for this berth.[1]

A dramatic pay and productivity deal has (1969) guaranteed a top pay of £39 a week to 240 dockers at a terminal berth in Millwall Dock in the port of London. Agreement has been reached between a shipping company and the White union. So far out are the terms of this contract that there is a genuine alarm by other employers at beating the pistol in a way that must set the pace for other agreements under phase 2. The high wages are inseparable from a more efficient system of working and the operation of a two-shift cycle. Good cargo handling drives out bad and, embarrassing as it may be, other employers will have to measure up to this "go it alone" movement.[2]

Training of Staff and Labour

When a port worker's skill did not rise above driving a crane or an electric truck, it was sufficient for the learner "to sit next to Nellie" and, finally, to be passed out by the dock engineer. Where machinery, the use of which involves the safety of other workers, is in question, it is right that

---

[1] "Should we then take a good look to the future and throw a certain amount of hereditary bias to one side and adopt an earnest view to arresting this position and what is more important, examining the possibilities of re-building" (Mr. T. Roffey, Transport Union official for the Tally Clerks in London).

[2] The agreement is based on productivity; the target for 1969 is three times that of 3 years ago with no extra labour.

it should not be used by uncertificated drivers. In the early years after the Second World War the introduction of mechanical equipment made it evident that a high standard of training would be necessary if the expensive new machines were to be preserved and made to work safely.

However small the port it should be possible to operate, or arrange access to, a training school where practical instruction in the safe use of forklift trucks and mobile cranes, particularly, can be given. If the number of men to be trained is small, the instructor can give personal help to each trainee. Similarly, some ground work in lighterage and export working should be possible. Demonstrations of heavy lift work, for instance, could be arranged with shipping companies. Much can be done with the written word when port workers are literate; this is assumed to be the case with the administrative staff. A profitable line is for the port authority to satisfy themselves that their higher executive staff not only understand the principles of port work but have an appreciation both of the work and its difficulties as done by the subordinate staff. It is a sound principle to adopt a method of breaking down the main operations of which cargo handling consists and to commit these to paper. When this is done, working instructions for the guidance of the staff can be prepared, printed, and issued, so that each member of the staff has his working "bible" and is familiar with the section that covers his activities. By this means uniformity of practice is obtained; this is of value in the interpretation of matters such as the regulations for the safe working of docks, ships, and their cargoes. Staff and labour can more readily be transferred throughout the undertaking when they react similarly to the same circumstances. A clearly understood code of duties and responsibilities for each division of the staff is valuable. When it has been assimilated, in conjunction with the regulations for the guidance of the staff, there is no excuse for action, or lack of action, that will involve the employer in losses, claims, or liabilities. It need hardly be stressed that regulations that are to be faithfully and intelligently observed can be compiled only after serious thought and by senior officers. Throughout all grades staff must have confidence that it is being asked to operate on instructions that are practical and which have been issued by practical officers.

With the prevailing problems of redundancy, the redeployment that this has already involved has stressed the need for retraining of the lesser number of men that the industry is shortly going to need. New cargo-handling processes require that thought be given constantly to the conversion of portworkers, whatever their trade, into highly trained and specialized operators.

"What do you know of [London] that only [London] know?" could well be adapted from Kipling. It was a well-known characteristic of the inter-war dock official that he was as well satisfied with the well-proved activities of his own port as he was ignorant and faintly contemptuous of those by which other ports strove and prospered. Now all that has changed. Training on a high level by the United Nations Technical Aid Bureau and the International Seminar on Port Management (in the hands of the Royal Netherlands universities), places on both of which are very much sought after, are supplemented by arrangements made between ports either in the same or in neighbouring countries. It is to the interest of every port that the ships which it handles should be equally well turned round elsewhere. Recently a team of dockers who were involved in disputes over the working of a new container berth were taken to Antwerp, Rotterdam, and Hamburg to see for themselves the calibre of the labour with whom their own port was in competition—a step more effective in restoring a sense of proportion than any amount of propaganda.

The technical press published in one's own language or in one from which appropriate articles can be translated is a valuable source of education for executives and should not be neglected.

Additional Notes

Chapter 6, page 91, par. 2. Reduction in dock labour. Dock labour fell in U.K. ports from 43,104 in 1969, to 38,923. In the port of London, from 21,066 to 18,259.

Page 97, par. 2. NDLB Annual Report for 1969 amended the largest age group to between 60–64 years—14·13 per cent of the total labour force. Only forty men were under 20.

Page 102, par. 1. Working Hours. The Port of Bristol Authority at their Avonmouth, Royal Edward Dock, now work round the clock.

CHAPTER 7

LABOUR II

A VAGUE humanitarian feeling can be traced in the writings of Victorian social historians on problems to do with the docks. Even their commendable liberal feelings could not suggest a better system than the one that for 150 years the whole country has deplored. The Port of London Act of 1908 and the official inquiry into dock conditions of 1920, better known as the Shaw Commission, both contained their well-meant platitudes on the need to replace casual by permanent labour. In the decade before the Second World War, negotiations for a permanent system did actually begin between employers and the unions, the latter accepting half of a 2s. (10p) a day rise demanded together with the promise to explore decasualization. The war put an end to these inconclusive discussions, and it was not until 30 years later that a full and comprehensive scheme was introduced. After 18 September 1967 no registered port worker was employed on other than permanent terms in the registered ports of the United Kingdom, and that by a single employer of his choice.

Decasualization has been so major a change in the conditions in which dock labour is now called upon to work that it has raised questions not many of which could have been anticipated prior to September 1967. The authors feel that it is worth while to deal with these briefly: were a similar system to be introduced into the ports of another country, one could be certain that although developments would not follow the same lines, the difficulties would, in the main, be similar. However, 3 years after the change came about a great deal remains to be done before the dock workers and the docks are in line in their work methods and in their construction with the latter half of the twentieth century.

Problems of Decasualization

No port operator was so simple as to imagine, despite national Dock labour boards and similar palliatives, that the change-over from a system based on casual employment would be done without grave labour troubles. The pre-war negotiations had foundered on the impracticability of settling the number of workers each port required. Whatever number was fixed in 1967 would be too many, because all registered port workers had a claim to permanency. Sacrifices were called for not only by the employers. The first snag lay in the absence of work for a proportion of the new permanent men. The whole pattern of each port suffered a jolt. Employers had always had their "choice" gangs of casual workers. They had learnt to manipulate the dock labour system so as to keep these in continuous work, and they did not hesitate to do this. The dock labour scheme of 1941 had been built up on the assumption, and no other was possible, that all port workers are equally good. It had taken the employers years, adequately helped by the dockers themselves, to demonstrate what all knew by instinct that some were better than others. Men had with the years settled down to do the jobs for which age, experience, and inclination had fitted them. Men who were used to good pay packets had now, in the interests of equality, to share work they had always regarded as their private domain with their fellow workers. In dock work there will always be good jobs as well as those from which, under piecework conditions, it is more difficult to extract a good return. On a wider scale the stevedores had to give up some of their traditional prestige. Certain areas in the port had always been regarded as "blue" territory; this was now invaded by "whites" who helped themselves to the plums. Reluctantly, because it was the only way the scheme could be worked, both unions agreed to a common register.

Redundancy

Concurrently with the arrival of the permanent job, to gain which six generations of dockers had fought and starved, came a threat to the job itself. The disquiet that had been felt by every thinking docker for two decades at the almost daily erosion in the demands of labour, found cogent expression in the McKinsey report prepared for the Docks Board of British Transport. In coming out openly with the verdict that 90 per cent of the present dock labour would be unwanted within a decade, it could not have chosen a less fortunate time. Co-operation by the employers in decasualization had been secured because of the early prospects of rationalizing the industry, for bringing cargo handling methods up to date and for progressively remodelling the work so that less men would be needed. All this, the need for which had been long accepted, was recognized in a report prepared by Lord Devlin. The programme to be negotiated, and which included shift working among other revolutionary proposals, came to be known, for convenience sake, as "Devlin Part 2". McKinsey was naturally played down by the employers—certain that labour was being asked to digest too much and that too quickly. Among themselves they thought that McKinsey would come about before the 10 years predicted. In a system of severance payments, mooted first at a figure of £600 but which reached £1800 in certain cases, men—some of whose grandfathers had fought the employers for 5 weeks for the "Dockers' tanner"—took this sum to leave the industry.[1] While the Government and the progressive politicians of both parties saw in decasualization an opportunity to right the wrongs of generations and to bring into the industry a happy state of co-operation, the men saw only one more shake-up of the cosy and conventional pattern of their daily lives.[2] It was change and a big change at that. Lord Devlin had remarked that the docker dislikes change even when it is for his own good. The immediate result was a strike, unofficial but none the less, solid. This lasted for 8 weeks and affected all the major ports in the United Kingdom. Decasualization got off to a bad start.

Phase 2

Discussion of the main clauses for an agreement to implement phase 2 eventually (April 1969) produced a simple formula. For a maximum guaranteed weekly wage of £33 10s. (£33.50) the three unions involved were to pledge their members to work two shifts daily in a working week consisting of 35 hours, to hold themselves available for week-end working, and at all times to be ready to work on any job to which they were directed (full flexibility and mobility). Important also, the unions were completely to observe the terms of this agreement, reverting to the conditions of the 1920s when the word of Ernest Bevin was his bond. Finally, there was to be a balanced labour force—all men were to be gainfully employed and "spelling" and other time-wasting practices were to cease. Were it possible to gain acceptance of these terms, a tremendous step forward would have

[1] The N.D.L.B. report of 1968 shows a net reduction in the Port Register of 1680 men.
[2] "We are experiencing a period now when everything is changing very rapidly. Not only do we have the impression that everything right down to its very foundations is changing, but we are scarcely given time to regain our breath after each innovation" (Mr. F. Suykens, Assistant General Manager, Port of Antwerp).

been taken. Progress has been slow.[1] Meanwhile the economic trend in dockland has overtaken the workers' reluctance to face facts. Unit loads, bulk cargoes, and containers with the altered pattern they have given to dock work, between them have closed the London and St. Katharine Docks, the Regents Canal Dock, and have threatened the large area traditionally devoted to loose timber handling—the Surrey Commercial Docks. Ports all over the world are being forced to take a serious look at their estates and to decide which docks have now been rendered out of date by the prevailing trends. Behind it all is the competition with the Benelux ports, which is unceasing and unrelenting.[2]

However, there were some who, after a year of decasualized labour, could claim that progress had been made and could point to new business in proof of this.[3] Certainly the most encouraging sign was the acceptance by a few of the more advanced of labour's dwindling legions of the package deal already described. The least encouraging was the willingness of the unions, while rendering lip-service to the idea, to use terminal agreements to demand a general pay agreement against the background of phase 2.

In many of the small ports there were real difficulties. Certain of these ports, by enlightened management and a reasonableness on labour's part that seems to diminish as ports get larger, had attained a prosperity in a couple of decades that London and Liverpool had sought unsuccessfully for more than 100 years. This was understandable, for growth in a port always produces its own problems. Decasualization was not easy to apply when dock work is seasonal and when it is sometimes a secondary occupation for local labour. In not all ports in the United Kingdom did the writ of the National Dock Labour Board run, and there were good reasons for this.

The major snag was, and continues to be, the embodiment of the two-shift system. It cannot be denied that domestic life has to be radically adjusted in a way far more drastic than that demanded by overtime working. Working habits that are the result of centuries of convention are disrupted. As with the arrangements that have to be made to deal with craft, rail

---

[1] In November 1969, after a postal ballet, the offer was turned down, involving the operation of the container berth at Tilbury Dock, which had been linked up with conditions elsewhere in the port of London.

[2] A serious warning to British dockers was given by a leading continental shipowner, Mr. Klaas de Waal of Amsterdam: "They have seen their diverted ships being happily handled by dockers who are just bemused by their British colleagues, attitude."

[3] On the other hand, it is asserted that up-to-date working in London would be delayed for another decade by "sheer stubbornness, conservatism, and shortsightedness."

wagons, and lorries loaded from ships working more than the one shift, so the movement of large bodies of workers call for alterations in public transport; peak hours no longer conform to custom and habit. Particularly are these changes emphasized in the lighterage industry. There are still, when two shifts are working, the same number of craft available to meet the needs of the port. There is, or should be, double the call on this number over a shorter period. Unless receiving wharves are willing—and there is no strong reason why they should be—to incur the additional cost of overtime, loaded craft will be left for working until the following day. This argument was brought up every time shift work had in the past been broached. It was a difficulty that had to be surmounted in such United Kingdom ports as were classed as overside because of the intense competition now being felt from the near continental ports. The urgency of the situation no longer permitted the problem to be met merely by a reiteration of old arguments. Discussions over phase 2 also brought out the lamentable condition of the means, in many ports, of communication between the two sides. It was still "them and us". Even officials of the union, if they attempted to put the employers' point of view, were dismissed as "them". In the summer of 1969, in a journal largely devoted to an unbiased presentation of facts about the ports, appeared a reference to the great Strike of 1889, wrongly thought to be dead and forgotten after 80 years. In the correspondence columns a letter referred to the "slave market, the Control Point in the Belfast Docks".[1] Throughout the talks that are still taking place (July 1969) there runs the thread of an agreement —and this is a very considerable step forward—that piecework and the gang system have had their day. Strict observance of the schedule will, it is increasingly seen, be futile as a weapon against competition from foreign ports,[2] as well as lesser competition from the ports of one's own country.

Nationalized Labour

It would have been strange if, in the searchings for a panacea for industrial troubles, labour had not put forward the nationalization of port labour as a means "to end inefficiencies and delays in cargo handling and help to cure the chaos of the casual system by making each port authority responsible for all port operations within its area, including stevedoring

[1] *The Port*, 5 June 1969.
[2] Ports such as Rotterdam have great natural advantages in the absence of tidal and locking problems.

etc." Although the ports' sub-committee of the Parliamentary Labour Party endorsed, in January 1969, this "commitment", a change in the ordinary dockers' outlook to work is not likely to be brought about by resolutions. Nor will it come by the inclusion in a proposed National Ports Authority, of which more will be said later, of 50 per cent of workers' representatives.

With the causes of redundancy worldwide and with decasualization a palliative or a deferment rather than a cure, it would be strange if there was not evidence that labour in other ports is not feeling the draught. Rotterdam, in the autumn of 1967 was emphatic that 3000–4000 dock workers would have to be laid off commencing forthwith, and in Dublin a substantial reduction was called for, a very serious matter in a port with so few alternative work opportunities. In the south of Italy a successful roll-on service for cars is run from Naples to Genoa and Palermo. The proprietors discovered a fact to which attention has already been drawn in these pages—that the owner of each car carried was also the shipper and the consignee of the cargo. Refusing to pay dockers for work they are no longer required to do and unable to reach agreement for compensatory pay for the small amount of general cargo their ships carry, they have transferred the service to nearby Castellamare-di-Stabia, adding to the large number of unemployed in the Naples area. In Belfast it is asserted that 400 men are now unwanted on the United Kingdom–Belfast run, and that a conversion to roll-on ships will make a further 100 redundant. As a natural consequence of the fewer number of men now needed to handle general cargo, there is a lesser demand for lighters. Unit loads and containers can be more quickly moved by road; they are independent of tidal delays, and drivers accept all-night working as normal.

Severance Payments

Lord Devonport, the leader of the London Port Employers during the major dock strike of 1912, said, in reply to Lloyd George's request that he should settle the strike, that those who were out could return at once— on the same terms as they went out. This reflected the basic feeling of the period; there was the job and the terms were x pence a day—you were free to take it or not; the employer was indifferent. Fifty years later the job, and the Rule Book that went with it, had come to be thought of in terms of property, the most valuable asset the worker had assumed for himself. It was one that would be surrendered only at a price. Therefore, having accepted this as a right, one of the more obvious ways of reducing a labour force was for the employer to pay a man to leave. The idea of severance pay was born and was first applied in the docks by the PLA a month after decasualization. Out of 785 of their dockers eligible for the scheme as then launched, 665 were willing to accept sums that varied from £200 to £600 to go; they remained entitled to any pension for which they had qualified. To many men, middle aged and with the sense to realize that the dwindling total of port work would be given to the younger men, it was a temptation to start up a business of their own. With some 1900 dockers eligible as the scheme developed and a normal annual outflow over the years of 8 per cent from the industry, the possibility of reducing the labour force now seemed practicable.

By July 1968 the scope of the scheme had been greatly widened despite some opposition from the unions who foresaw that a payment—the equivalent of a year and a half's pay—would in many cases be squandered long before that time. Agreement was reached that enabled men with more than 28 years' service to qualify for the upper limit of £1800. It was predicted that 4500 PLA and 18,000 men working for other port employers would now be eligible. Some 200 lightermen had also left what some considered to be fast becoming a dying industry.

In May 1969 severance was put on a sound footing by a government loan of £3 million. It was ordered that the National Dock Labour Board should take over the running of the scheme, the remaining money of the £7 million estimated to be needed, being provided by a $2\frac{1}{2}$ per cent levy on the employers' wage bills. A reassuring feature was the inclusion of the chronically sick and those incapable of doing a full day's work. By the end of June of the same year, following a survey of labour requirements made by the board, an initial estimate of a 10 per cent cut was made following the next phase of the severance scheme.

Pensions

To aid the prevalent tendency, the compulsory retiring age has (June 1969) been lowered from 68 to 65 years; each man's weekly contribution has gone up to 10s. (50p) from the previous 5s. (25p).

Amenities

A general agreement that the standard of amenities is deplorably low in the docks has done little to resolve problems of responsibility for providing them. Employers are reluctant to build, equip, and staff modern canteens which will be enjoyed by general users of the docks, bearing in mind that such amenities will always need to be subsidized. However, the port authority in London have embarked on the building of comprehensive "amenity blocks" containing a tea bar, mess room, lockers for dockers' clothes, showers, and lavatories; the buildings are centrally heated.

Loss of Business

Inevitably the trend in the past two decades has been to reduce the demand for labour. The tide has swept in with increasing force and no sign can be discerned of its yet having reached its full state, let alone setting in on an ebb. No single agent has done more to make dock workers redundant than the container and its companions, the unit load, and the bulk cargo. No single agent has done more to make the introduction of the container inevitable than the dock worker. To devise means of reducing the call on dock labour was the obvious reaction of the commercial community—the chief sufferers from the anarchic condition in the docks, in the years immediately following the Second World War, when "either, else" dominated the work. The container is winning and labour is fighting a losing battle. Instead of guarding jealously the moiety of work that remains, labour has, since decasualization, given the impression of having gone out of its way to jettison even this.[1] It is a feature of the period that neither the layman nor the Press can comprehend. Foreign ports have been quick to take the traffic that a suicidal policy—if it can be called a policy—has thrown at them.[2] The social historian of the future will regretfully record that in the art of self-destruction the porcine population of Gadara, in the first century, had nothing to teach the British docker of the twentieth century.[3] Those who profess to understand something of the way he reaches his conclusion may find it possible to follow his reasoning. On all sides he

[1] As an instance, the United Steamship Company of Denmark, after 50 years trading with London, is to concentrate on roll-on unit-load ships at east coast ports.
[2] An American expert speaking at Melbourne charged British dock labour with economic treason, adding: "When a nation is fighting for its life in the war for economic trade, the social structure and government cannot long tolerate those who would sabotage these efforts."
[3] Pilferage among consignments of fine ware from Italy having now reached 8 per cent of the cargo, the importers are bringing in their merchandise overland via Dover—at one-third of the sea cost.

sees his work disappearing.[1] To show his disapproval of the terms being discussed under phase 2, he brings out his tried and trusted weapon—the unofficial strike, not understanding that a bludgeon of this type is power-less against economic forces. He knows the position is desperate, and his reaction to recommendations made under Phase 2 is not to accommodate himself to new conditions of working but to attempt to make use of the concessions that they demand as bargaining counters. If this policy means that work leaves the port, it cannot be helped—it is a "calculated gamble". To cope with the tremendous problem that the dock industry faces in every port of any size in the world and in varying degrees, requires a standard of reasoning and co-operation that the antecedents of port labour do nothing to promise. The outlook as expressed from Rotterdam may well be correct: "I believe that containers are not just a development of the old business of stevedoring, *it's becoming a completely new industry* and we're determined to lead it." With an industry so traditionally bound to the past there is neither the ability nor the desire from labour to look at problems in so inconvenient a light. A brief survey of some of the actions taken by port labour in their fight over phase 2 and the results to the time of writing (November 1969) may be of interest to ports in other countries where they may have to face the same international problem. Only by looking at the struggle against the background of phase 2 can it be understood.

London

The working of container berths constructed for the Australian container trade at Tilbury Dock was covered by a team agreement made locally. Before this could be put into operation the union forbad it. They took the stand that it was far too valuable a weapon and it should be kept for negotiations for labour throughout the port during the coming phase 2 discussions. The result has been that containers for Australia are being shipped via small English ports to Antwerp where the new container ships

[1] *Technical and Social Change in the World's Ports*, a report published in July 1969 by the International Labour Office, deals with the long shadow cast from London to Los Angeles by the container and the mechanization of cargo handling methods. "While the extent of the problem created by new methods and equipment should not be exaggerated, there is enough substance in the predictions made as to the impact on labour to cause anxiety among dockers about their future job prospects. These fears will also cause the workers to cling to practices designed to keep up the numbers employed on a job beyond the level really required. The whole issue of restrictive practices is, of course, directly related to the fear of under-employment."

are loading. One thousand three hundred containers were so diverted for the first ship.[1]

"Rotterdam is being allowed to stage a perfect dress rehearsal of the situation it will fight with all the weapons to make permanent, ludicrously helped by dockers at Tilbury, who, while refusing to handle the ships themselves, are working the feeder ships that serve them."[2]

The trade envisaged from New Zealand to London will be diverted to Southampton if a satisfactory agreement to use London cannot be reached.[3] There is a substantial import trade in meat, dairy produce, and fruit, and this will be jeopardized unless the container problem can be solved.

Timber ships destined to be discharged at the newly constructed berth at Tilbury Dock are being delayed over disputed conditions; the delay is costing the owners £1000 per day. Their diversion to trouble-free ports is envisaged.

Mark Brown's Wharf, an old-fashioned riverside wharf on the Thames, has had continuous trouble over phase 2—a stoppage every 3 days, as conditions there have been described. It has now closed down. This was due to the diversion of the ships of Polish Ocean Lines to the trouble-free port of Ipswich. The men's immediate reaction was a demonstration march to the Polish Embassy in London. Here they were given a polite reception but no action followed. Since 1967 it is alleged that 123 stoppages have occurred there. Shippers' reaction is: "Your charges have gone up but your service has come down."

Hays Wharf, the major wharf in a large Thames group, was shut down on 12 December 1969. Since decasualization, 60 per cent of their trade has been lost.

Fennings Wharf. Dutch ships using this terminal have been diverted to another part of the Port of London; once the warehoused cargo has been delivered the wharf may close.[4]

London is by no means the only troubled port in the United Kingdom. Liverpool has been bedevilled by unofficial stoppages. It has been said that a strike a day can be predicted. Despite a shortage of labour there, three

[1] The ease with which cargoes can be and are being re-routed to trouble-free ports is overlooked by dockers.
[2] *The Times.*
[3] Container services to the Far East will now operate from Southampton.
[4] The large-scale on which riverside wharfs in London are being closed down is further reducing the work available to the lighterage trade. A serious feature of this, although not given publicity, is the large number of wharf staff, some after 40 years' service, who are now redundant.

ships recently stopped work over a minor dispute. Tariff charges have been increasing; the Mersey Docks and Harbour Board attribute the loss of £1·2 million during 1968 to a disruptive element in the port. The pattern that the stoppages take, apart from 1-day token strikes, is for all ships to cease work if a dispute over a minor matter, such as the allowance to be paid for dirty cargo, is not quickly settled. By this is meant that the employer is expected to give way. During December 1968, eighty sailings were affected and the port is getting a reputation for unreliability. Unless a guarantee of uninterrupted discharge can be given, a shipping line taking bananas to Liverpool will send no more ships there. In July 1969 all container traffic in and out of Liverpool, which in 1968 amounted to more than 100,000 units, was temporarily "blacked" after a dispute over the employment of dockers at the nearby storage depot.[1]

Nearby *Manchester*, until recently one of the most reliable and efficient of United Kingdom ports, has been plagued with 1-day token strikes, ostensibly to obtain better conditions for work under phase 2. In the east coast port of *Hull*, owing to the lesser demand for labour, one dock (part of the port), was closed in August 1969 and a further part of the estate may be filled in to make a reception area for containers.

Even the municipally run port of *Bristol* is not without its troubles. The trade, now 50 years old and producing six ships each season for the discharge there of Jaffa citrus fruit, has, due to an overtime ban been diverted to Cardiff.

This is indeed a sorry catalogue of self-destruction whether the docker calls it a calculated gamble or not. Official figures for the number of days lost in British ports in 1967, the year of decasualization, was 606,000—all unofficial. This does not and cannot take account of days lost by the dozens of ancillary traders that depend on normal working in the ports—if "normal working" as a term can now have much significance. One can conclude this brief survey by two observations made by parties that are certainly, and have every reason to be, interested in the curious conduct of the British docker. "Thank you, England", said a Rotterdam Harbour official, briefly saluting in a gesture of contempt for British dockers. He was probably grateful for the extra business they are pushing his way. He was also puzzled, as indeed most people are. He spoke knowing that shipowners all over the world were reading a shrewdly timed circular

---

[1] In December 1969 agreement was reached with Liverpool dockers, "the men had got to protect themselves", to handle containers.

which said that Rotterdam's stable labour relations, whereby risks of strike delays are minimal, was the reason for its rise as Europe's container capital. More than a million tons of cargo was lost to London last year because of shipping lines' exasperation with labour relations. It won't come back.[1]

The message handed to labour representatives sent from London to see for themselves how traffic diverted from London was being handled at Antwerp, was simple and to the point: "we will handle as many container ships as you care to send us."

However, it is not the intention to represent ports of the United Kingdom, and particularly London, as being prone whilst those in other countries have been immune from the fear that containerization will affect their job prospects for the future. *This is far from being the case.*

From the recent International Labour Office report *Technical and Social Change in the World's Ports* (referred to in footnote on p. 118) it is clear that no country of any maritime importance has been exempt from the wave of unrest that has followed the introduction of phase 2 in the United Kingdom and the equivalent attempts at dock modernization made elsewhere.

Gothenburg has now reached agreement on two-shift working. The port of New York has a long record of strife, despite a scheme for decasualization that goes back to 1954. There was trouble over containers in 1958 and it was not until 1965 that the union accepted reductions in the strength of basic gangs. In nearby St. Lawrence ports, labour disputes over this issue go back several years, culminating in the serious strikes of May and June 1966. Tally clerks in Australian ports have been on strike, and dockers in Venezuela have refused to work container berths. From London to Tokyo, from Melbourne to New York, dockers share the same fear that new methods will mean redundancy, and in this they are correct.

Problems of the Future

At no time in the history of the world's ports has the industry been beset by so many major problems. Some of them are capable of solution internally, given goodwill. Others are not so capable—they seem in fact insoluble and[2] one of these is the intrusion of air freight. Ten years ago

---

[1] From an article "Rotterdam loves our dockers" published in *The Observer* and quoted in *The Port*, 5 June 1969.

[2] The large increases given to labour recently and in particular where team work has guaranteed these is causing unrest among executive and operative staff whose rewards are often less than the labour they supervise.

shipping and port circles had not reached the stage of taking carriage of goods by air at all seriously. It was true that a few tons of cargo, valuable enough to stand the necessarily high freight charges, was being carried. Today a shipper with a few tons of electronic cargo wanted, say, in Lisbon, can tender this at a United Kingdom airport in the morning and it will be in his customer's hands later in the day. Compare this with the leisurely process of sending the same cargo to a port. Here it will remain in the export shed for a few days awaiting shipment. This is followed by a voyage still dependent on weather, to be followed later by the leisurely process of discharge into a shed. There may be delay whilst the national Customs clear the goods, until eventually a lorry arrives to take delivery. What in air traffic is counted in hours is reckoned by ships in days.

This is a brief account of the vicissitudes, frustrations, and minor triumphs that have followed decasualization in the United Kingdom; they are by no means yet settled.

Additional Notes

Chapter 7, page 112, par. 1. Reduction of dock force. Dockers are leaving the industry (July 1970) at the rate of 80–100 men per week.

Page 113, par. 1. Closure of Surrey Commercial Docks, London. This has been agreed for 1970.

Page 115, par. 3. NDLB paid out more than £5 million in Severance Payments in 1969.

Page 119, par. 1. Container berth at Tilbury. This squabble was not settled until June 1970, to cease work again with the national dock strike of July 1970.

Page 119, par. 6. Hays Wharf. The closure of this wharf got rid of over 400 men.

CHAPTER 8

GENERAL-CARGO WORK

Introduction

Before moving on to the engrossing topic of containers and the problems they are raising, it will be worth while to look at the improvements that have been taking place in the turnround of general-cargo ships and to examine some of the causes. Spectacular out-turns are to be expected in the discharge of bulk cargoes and of ships containing one type only of unit loads. Under the aspects of export and import working, including barge, road, and rail, we shall trace and explain how gradually the gang-hour figure on general cargo has crept up. While labour troubles can be sure of front-page notices in the national press, consistently good out-turns do not make news.

Changes Ancillary to Mechanization

Forklift trucks and mobile cranes, particularly among items introduced for the mechanical handling of cargo, demand hard gangways, concrete quays, suitably sized doors in sheds, and a number of improvements that, collectively, have put the pre-1939 transit shed into the category of second-class buildings. The new type of shed has included useful balconies on which cargo can be landed or shipped from, protection from rain being given to men working below in the case of the obtruded type. The clutter of small buildings that were, it might almost be said, encouraged to find a home in the valuable area of the transit shed have been banished. A realization that every square yard of a dock building is there to earn money will prevent their ever returning. The many gangways that were meant to avoid payment for extra trucking are, with the use of forklift trucks, only an unhappy memory, as is the large number of shed doors, each of which led to one more gangway and more space that could not be used for storage.

Increasing Use of Pallets

It is indeed difficult to speak highly enough of the role that the pallet has come to play in port working. Some historically minded port operators see the pallet as having been used in building the Pyramids but, failing the forklift truck, it was more probably a primitive tray that subsequently developed into the highly effective cargo-landing board used so extensively in the inter-war years. Without the forklift truck, by the use of which the unit of cargo can be transported and piled intact, the landing board remains a tray adapted for slinging. This is exactly the shape taken by the stevedore's pallet, devised and first used on exports in 1947.

There are so many uses to which pallets can be put by port authorities, from ship discharge to the internal transfer of warehoused cargo, that it is well worth the time to study the type that their prevailing cargo dictates. As an example, the first shipment of tea was made early in 1966, on pallets.[1] A port specializing in tea should provide itself with pallets of a size to cope with the modal unit, the chest of tea.

Every time that cargo is put loose into a barge, labour is used to make up and to sling the sets, receive these in the craft, break them down, and stow each package separately. The process is reversed when the barge is discharged. When the port authority has its own lighterage department, work can be speeded up by instituting a system of palletized cargo handling. There is, naturally, a considerable transfer of general cargo by barge between Rotterdam and Amsterdam; a conventionally loaded barge made the trip once or one and a half times a week. A barge loaded solely with pallet units can load and discharge in one day with reduction from four to two in the number of men doing the work. Palletized cargoes discharged from ships—and this covers pallets loaded by stevedores in the hold—can expect a gang-hour tonnage of 40 tons in place of the 25 tons normal for loose cargo. Two men to receive the pallet on the quay, plus one forklift truck driver, have replaced the gang of a dozen or more truckmen required for loose cargo. There are similar advantages to be gained in palletizing cargo for road transport.

If every bag of raw material in a consignment has to be weighed singly for trade or Custom's purposes, there is no reason why this service should not be speeded by port authorities palletizing the loads. Prior to the

---

[1] The tea trade are now considering altering the present size of tea chests to a modular size of one of the ISO standard pallets.

importation of sugar in bulk, millions of bags for storage were weighed singly, each bag being deposited on a deadweight scale by a truckman. Later it was found possible to weigh sets of Cuban sugar as they were landed from the ship, and this was an improvement on a process inconceivably tedious, but hallowed as a custom of the port. When orders are received, prior to landing, for a parcel to be weighed, the pallets that will be used in the operation can be selected, numbered, and each one weighed. If the pallets are metal it is necessary only to weigh one, but wooden pallets do vary with temperature and humidity. Each pallet load can be deposited on the pan of the deadweight or mechanical scale and over the run of the parcel, weighing is extraordinarily accurate.

Although the size of the stevedore pallet has been standardized, there is nothing to prevent port authorities from using pallets of a size designed on a modal basis. Containers can be quickly loaded with cases or cartons and pallets of a size that will allow two at a time to cover the floor of the container. So favourable have been the results obtained in this way that advice to likely users of pallets is now available from firms who have gained experience in improving output. Loading the palletized cargo through side doors of general cargo ships is a case in point. Where fragile cargo, such as baskets of vegetables or fruit has to be tendered to the ship for loading, a very large set can be built up on a pallet and slung aboard without damage; this is done by a stretcher designed to the dimensions of the load.

There will always be argument between the exponents of containers and unitized pallet loads. It has been demonstrated that container ships are economic when the voyage is more than 3000 miles, and that for less than this distance pallet ships have been successful. In the case of a ship of this kind on a Far Eastern run it is claimed that she will load as much cargo in Sydney in 1 day as a general-cargo vessel will in 10; labour costs have been drastically cut. Pallet ships are the less ostentatious but effective relation of the container ship. The highly disruptive effects of the container ship, particularly as it gets bigger, on our present distributive system, might be effectively met by the increasing use of pallet ships.

Expendable pallets are not likely to be extensively used by port authorities, although considerable progress has been made in specialized trades; useful pallets are now being manufactured from paper. Extensive research has been made into types and their usage, and this is available.[1] Not only are

[1] D. Wilson, *The Use of Expendable Pallets*, Merseyside Productivity Association.

forklift trucks becoming as essential on board ship as the ship's winches, but a recently built Swedish roll-on ship has included a 10-ton capacity hydraulic lift for forklift trucks and pallet loads.

Tallying

In an age of computers and electronics it is difficult to accept that no effective substitute has yet been evolved for the visual tallying of general cargo. The small number of packages in the average bill of lading, the peculiarities of the cargo, the liability either through frail, unsuitable, or insufficient packaging for damage to occur, plus the suspicion that either by design or accident there will be a shortage in the out-turn, all these reasons have conspired to preserve a system of checking cargo that is not substantially different from that used by the English poet, Geoffrey Chaucer, when he tallied cargo for his royal master Edward III, more than 500 years ago. Meat discharged on the conveyors, carton traffic in bananas, and in fact any homogeneous cargo, will lend itself to one of the automatic methods of recording out-turn. With bulk cargo, electronic weighing devices will give the shipping company and the importer reliable informa- tion. It is, however, the small bill of lading—and these constitute the bulk of general cargo carried today—that has ensured the continued employ- ment of tally clerks. Like so many customs of the port, a bold and deter- mined onslaught will cause it to topple. Many of the world's ports have abolished tallying. The pessimist who predicted that an avalanche of claims would immediately follow, has been everywhere confounded. Such claims as have been established have amounted to a tithe only of the present high cost of tallying. Even the defenders of the present system do not pretend that it is, nor ever can be, 100 per cent accurate. The more the effort to make it so, the more delay there is to the movement of cargo. It is a port practice that will disappear with the container and the unit load. It will persist, however, because of the grip that the practice has in all the major ports, reinforced by the disinclination of port authorities to add to potential labour troubles.

If tallying as a dock practice is to be continued, is there not a better way of doing it than the traditional squinting by a clerk at sets swinging from the crane hook? The East African Railways and Harbours thought so and invented the "in-stack" method which has been copied in South African ports. Basically it substitutes the inaccurate and often ineffective attempts to tally cargo while in motion by a more leisurely and certainly more accurate counting of cargoes after they have been landed. The system has worked well for some years.

Sorting at Landing

Just as there is no revenue for the port authority in tallying, so the practice of sorting cargo to bill of lading marks is unremunerative. In fact, sorting to both marks and grades is the main enemy of mechanization. Only when sorting has been eliminated can mechanical handling function. Citrus fruit was for years a difficult commodity to handle because of the excessive marks the cases carried—in some instances every few hundred boxes of oranges grown on separate estates advertised this fact by separate marking. After discussion with importers a simple code was substituted; it became easier to identify consignments of similar grades and the process was mechanized. Once again a resolute approach by the port authority demolished a custom of the port.

Fragile Cargoes

Efforts to speed the handling of certain cargoes—fresh eggs particularly —were thwarted so long as consignments were treated as general cargo. Where the traffic is constant it is worth while to have it palletized in specially designed pallets that enable a sizeable unit load to be lifted safely and without damage.

Intermittent Work

In the past, local shed staff have worked out a liaison system with importers so as to keep delivery gangs permanently at work. This has been a sensible, if somewhat empiric, answer to the problem. Following a survey of dock deliveries, a major port in the United Kingdom has recently instituted a pre-booking system by which hauliers can leave a given number of trailers on one day at a berth and collect them with mechanical horses on the following day. As the work of loading goes on during the night, the drivers' time is not wasted watching the loading; the frequent complaints of waste of the time of drivers have been avoided. It is just one more custom of the port—the right of a driver to apply for a load at his own convenience—that has quietly disappeared.

Special Gear

Even the oldest, the most primitive, but still often the most effective piece of cargo-handling gear, the sling for bag cargo has been improved as the result of recent research. An alternative to the pallet or the bound unit load is the sling unit, particularly for use with paper bags when consignments of these alternate or are stowed in the ship in conjunction with parcels in bulk. A type of sling has now been produced that is returnable in those staple trades that work on a recognized shuttle service. The ease with which slings can be returned as compared with pallets or containers is a factor in the preference shown by shippers for this means of unitizing a load. Specially designed nylon cloth and terylene webbing slings are now produced for handling paper bags in sets—up to twenty bags at a time.

Grabs for varied-bulk cargoes such as cake and small stones, as well as magnet types for scrap metal and claw grabs for pit props, are now available. After many unsuccessful experiments, the grab adopted for the kangaroo-type quay crane has not been surpassed for the discharge of that most difficult bulk cargo, raw sugar. Grabs for general bulk can be fitted to a certain type of container crane, both for loading and discharge, so that when not in use for containers the berth can be gainfully employed for bulk.

In countries where wharf congestion is a real threat and where development space is non-existent, or mountains have to be moved to make it, it may be possible to berth, say, a container ship that needs considerable wharf space, in the stream and to discharge the cargo in to self-propelled trains of large lighters that are permanently linked in groups of three. Several of these trains can work a shuttle service between the anchorage in the stream and a depot out of town where there is sufficient space to handle the cargo. It is claimed by the Australian Stevedoring Industry Authority, where this system is advocated, that three trains of lighters would carry the equivalent of twenty-five rail trains. Lighter trains could profitably be used for other unitized cargoes, particularly packaged timber. Ferro-cement lighters which proved their worth in the Second World War are recommended because the first costs, also the maintenance, are less than for conventional craft.

Only the spread of containers will settle, by making it out of date, the argument on the advantages of the quay crane over the ship's winches.

This is not the place to chronicle the see-saw struggle that has gone on since the nineteenth century, how, from the early fixed jib hydraulic pioneers, there has developed the electric level luffing crane, and how from the deck-installed "roundabout", emitting steam from its many valves, came the silent electric winch. From many years' experience it can be said that the best equipment is the one that will do the job the most cheaply and effectively. In this assessment the type of crane cycle required is a major factor. An old-fashioned 30 cwt fixed jib hydraulic, with its relatively quick slewing, can transfer a surprisingly high tonnage from ship to shore when all the cargo is under plumb and can be received at the side of the ship on electric trucks. On the other hand, if cargo has to be "searched for" in the wings of a lower hold, the derricks have greater flexibility than the crane, even with its gooseneck luffing facilities. Again, the kangaroo crane, dropping its grab load of sugar into its "pouch" with a minimum of slewing (already referred to), cannot be rivalled by a union purchase rig that must work within a transverse and inflexible path.

The solution may in fact be found in the use of high mounted mobile cranes that can plumb the ship's hold from the quay. These have the great merit that they can be moved round from one job to the next, thus avoiding the capital loss caused by equipment unused when berths are unoccupied.

In some ports with restricted water space there is difficulty in housing, by rafting, imports of large mahogany logs used in the fast-growing plywood industry. This is a further instance of a very partial use being made of storage space—in this case the dock water used only as to its surface area. There is nothing to prevent the piling of floated timber, the height of the pile being limited to the depth of the water area selected. This could be, ideally, a disused dry dock such as exists in many ports where dry-dock accommodation for small vessels is no longer fully used. After de-watering the dock it can be filled with logs; by using a mobile crane to lift these from the raft moored by the dry-dock gates, each log can be placed on the pile being formed in the dock. A start can be made by cramming the dock, filled with water, with as many of the rafts as possible, cutting the head and breast ropes and allowing the logs to sink to the floor when the dry dock is de-watered. By slinging wire nets, of the ship's side kind, across the width of the dry dock, stowages for separate merchants can be preserved. Deliveries can be made by mobile crane and the logs re-rafted if the consignees have waterside premises; alternatively, they can be delivered to craft or road vehicle. Some ten times the tonnage of logs can be housed in a dry dock as on a water area of comparable size.

Exports

The major change in the handling of exports by port authorities since 1945 has been the application of the principle of the larger cargo unit which has enabled loose exports to be mechanized. Prior to the introduction of the system, a gang of six men could be relied upon to strike and to pass into the shed, with hand trucks, some 50 tons per day. Work normally continued until 7 p.m., and delays of many hours to lorries was accepted as unavoidable. The modern system is very simple. One mobile crane loads a dock pallet direct from the lorry parked some yards from the rear of the shed. As each pallet is completely loaded, it is run into the shed by a forklift truck where a succession of palletized exports 20 ft high is piled to ports. Subsequently, as the loading stevedores call for the export cargo it is run out under plumb of the crane or the ship's gear. Only when the pallet load is placed in the hold stow are the loose packages taken off. Experiments with expendable pallets lead one to hope that it will be possible to leave these intact in the ship's hold. With a gang of three men an output of some 300 tons for an 8-hour working day on striking and shedding exports is now normal, and delays to lorries are disappearing.

The importance of making up small units of export cargo is realized, but progress in this direction has been hindered by a number of practical difficulties. Consignments amounting to less than 3 tons (and their number is considerable) can be dealt with at central receiving depots which are now beginning to function. They have eliminated some of the delays caused by having to cater for small parcels that can be conveniently presented to the ship in one or more barge loads already consolidated to ports. In the port of Hamburg 7–8 million small packages of high-grade export goods are received, stored, and consolidated for over 19,000 sailings in a year.

The difficulty of regulating the reception of export cargoes when presented in full lorry loads has, in the past, led to delays in unloading and congestion on the dock roads and also on the approach roads to the port. Instead of moving slowly along the queue that built up at the rear of each export berth, the driver can now report to one of the lorry parks that serve each of the main export areas in a modern port (Fig. 22). The traffic lanes within the park are allocated according to the loading vessels. The driver is called by loudspeaker when a telephone message from the shed concerned tells the lorry park officer that the berth can receive a further batch of lorries. As a modern lorry park will hold 350 vehicles, this number can be taken off the dock roads. Their contents can be looked at selectively, cargo of a like nature can be called forward instead

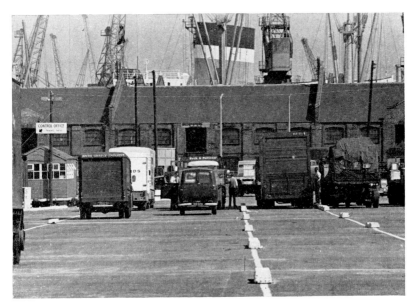

FIG. 22. Lorry park for exports, Royal Docks, London. (By courtesy of PLA.)

of cargo of very varied kinds arriving indiscriminately at the doors of the export shed. Drivers can be warned when there will be delay and can take their meals, knowing that they will not be called within the time that this will take. A further valuable step in controlling the reception of export cargo has also been made possible—the lorry pre-booking scheme. As far back as 1947 a scheme was put forward in a major port that would have given the port authority the same measure of shed control with exports arriving as with imports landed. At the time shippers had not learnt, with the experience so hardly gained since, that co-operation with the port authority will always pay dividends. At certain docks shippers can now "book" time, greatly to their saving. When this is done by all the principal shippers, and they have not been slow to see the advantages, an even flow of exports to a "large loader" can almost be guaranteed and the alternate slack and congested periods which wasted the time of labour and lorry drivers, avoided. Although off-loading times cannot be guaranteed, preference is naturally given to unloading "booked" vehicles.

Encouragement has also been given by the modern port, in the form of cheaper terminal charges, to those shippers who have contrived to unitize their export packages. An outstanding example is the bundling of motor-car tyres, for long a tiresome and space wasting traffic. A 20-ton capacity box car, when filled with loose tyres, would not carry more than 8 tons. By using a machine to compress twenty tyres at a time in a horizontal bundle, space is saved, several bundles at a time can be lifted by forklift truck or piled from a pyramidical base; the bundle can be handled as a taut consignment instead of an uncontrollable medley of individual tyres.

In the heyday of conventional cargo handling, export packages that weighed more than the ship's gear or the quay crane could handle had to be placed on board by a heavy-lift floating derrick. This was a slow, time-wasting job; work in the hold had to be suspended whilst a package weighing perhaps 20 tons was angled into position by a cumbersome derrick. By installing a heavy mobile crane at a convenient barge berth, all lifts beyond the ship's capacity can be unloaded from lorry or rail, placed on the quay or put directly into craft (when it is possible to make up a full barge load), and this is dispatched alongside at a time suitable to the shipping company. The waste of time associated with the intermittent handling of heavy lifts has now been avoided. Some use has been made of barges for loading exports direct from rail wagons so as to avoid congestion in the sheds. Similarly, it has been found possible to receive and to ship off exports from an upper floor of a modern transit shed, thus adding to the space available for receiving export cargoes.

Lighterage

The main enemy of port working is congestion. This happens when the number of packages is greater than the labour available can pick up and put down during the hours that it is willing to work. It is often brought about because cargo is handled solely across the quays. This is the way that the primitive port commences to do its work and it continues in this way after the amount of business has increased to such an extent that demands a basic re-examination of the port's methods. Often the amount of space ashore is limited by the geography of the country—mountains come down to the sea or urban development has taken up any available ground.[1] In this case the situation must be boldly tackled by restoring to the alternative outlet for cargo—the barge. In estuarial ports there is much overside traffic, and this method is used extensively by receivers with waterside premises. Railways often take their cargo overside for transhipment at a waterside rail depot. In ports where over 50 per cent of the cargo in either direction can be lightered, congestion is a diminishing spectre. The formation by a port authority of its own lighterage department is a bold move against congestion; it demands capital, building of the right number of barges of a suitable type, providing tugs, lightermen and staff, and the overcoming of prejudice among receivers over double handling. It is obviously more expensive to take goods meant for landing into craft and to deliver these via a lighterage berth elsewhere in the port, but if it will avoid congestion it is very much worth doing.[2] During the working of a large general-cargo ship there will be many opportunities to use a flexibility that this alternative outlet provides. Needless to say, cargo intended for the lighterage berth should be palletized within the hold at discharge.

External lighterage is suffering from the competition of road and rail; the part that it will play in container traffic has not yet been determined.[3] There are arguments against further increasing the burden on congested roads; the open river has advantages that lighter owners are not slow to point out. Looking over their shoulders, they are aware of the movement to bring loaded barges, in the form of the largest of general cargo units, directly into ports. They have already considered the possibility of their own port being used as a terminal for ships of the LASH type.[4] Some rationalization in the absorption of small firms has taken place, and steps have been taken to tackle that ancient bugbear and a most hardy custom

[1] In the port of Bar, in southern Yugoslavia, the mountain side has been cut away to make possible the building of a quay. This could be adapted, by building a road down the slope, for a gravity feed for bulk bauxite, loading into vessels lying alongside. In this way the mountain is being made use of.
[2] See Appendix I on the formation of an internal lighterage system.
[3] A weekly barge service for containers operates on the Rhine from Amsterdam to Basle, via Mannheim, Karlsruhe, and Strasbourg.
[4] The "Seabee" barge with its parent ship comes within the same category of cargo transporter.

of the port—the puny size of the general-cargo barge. This has hardly altered in the port of London since A.D. 1514. Ignoring the effectiveness of the Rhine barges and persisting in inflicting the handicap of constant barge replacement around a busy overside ship was a practice to be found not only in British ports. At last convention has been discarded and a start has been made to match the modern grain terminal in the port of London with a 1000-ton bulk grain barge. This will hold four times the cargo of the larger Thames craft. The amount of time lost in taking out the full barge and replacing with the empty one, the tug power, and the labour involved in getting barges in and out of an enclosed dock has been a disgrace to modern cargo handling. One dock that boasted for years of handling 500 barges a day during the peak season did not realize that this was a reproach to the efficiency of the trades concerned.

As an aid to efficiency there are now barges built to carry round logs and to dump these through stern doors. It is of some interest to note that the sailing barge, long a prominent feature on English tidal waters in Great Britain, is now represented by one survivor of a one-time proud fleet. This does not mean that they are not of importance in the ports of many countries, particularly in the Far East. Without the powered barges, run on family lines, the business of Hong Kong would soon grind to a stop over its limited run of quays.

The usefulness of barges as an outlet for cargo intended for quay delivery cannot be over-emphasized; in no circumstances should they be allowed to function as temporary warehouses. Their turnround is second only to that of ships.

Rail Working

The arguments that have been put forward in favour of a port authority making itself responsible for internal lighterage apply equally to internal rail work.[1] During the time that rail was predominant over road, and this lasted for many decades, most berths were rail served. The very up-to-date methods that the railways have evolved for handling containers and the like traffic has hit back at the roads. Small consignments can now be delivered by contractors' lorries from the rail head to the berth, involving the minimum use of the public roads.

For many decades port operators were in favour of delivering cargo

[1] See Appendix II for a suggested organization of a rail department by a port authority.

direct from the ship to rail wagons; likewise they went to great trouble to ship exports directly from the quay. Berths built between the wars were equipped with several lines of rails for a mythical traffic that seldom materialized. It is true that parcels of barbed wire and scrap iron—exceptional parcels of this kind—were economic if handled directly. Like many other of the good ideas that have turned into "follies" in our ports, the advocates of direct handling visualized continuous work, day after day, with standard-sized gangs, the saving on which would amply pay for the cost of working rail traffic. Frozen and chilled meat, a high proportion of which is delivered to rail, soon demonstrated that direct quay working would lead directly to congestion and to the stopping of the ship with every shunt. In addition, movement of the trucks stopped work at holds where general cargo was being discharged. Before long rail wagons were banished to lines at the shed rear, where alternative standings allowed for shunting. A recently built shed in the port of London was equipped with rails at the rear of the shed only.[1]

General Improvements

Every go-ahead port has sought to improve its cargo-handling methods in accordance with the type of cargo in which it specializes. As an example, in a port that exports steel in long lengths, sheds have been built with sliding roofs out of which bundles of steel can be shipped direct. The standard-sized side door on the open rail wagon that was satisfactory in the days of single-bag loading from hand trucks has been replaced by wide side doors which made loading by forklift trucks practical. Hinged and sliding roofs on wagons have also taken advantage of the benefits that the single-pull hatch covers have given to the cargo ship. There is, indeed, scope for adapting mechanization to all stages in cargo handling; this is a field where helpful suggestion is more likely to come from the operatives in the shed than the planners in their offices.

Additional Note
    Chapter 8, page 135, par. 2. Railway closures. As from 1st May 1970 the PLA closed its rail service to individual berths.

---

[1] No. 4 shed at the Royal Victoria Dock. The most recently built sheds at Tilbury Dock have rail lines only at the rear.

CHAPTER 9

THE CONTAINER TRAFFIC I

Introduction

The search for the larger cargo unit has achieved its object in the container. The bag, bale, or wooden case that owed its shape and its weight to the limitations imposed by manual handling, is giving way to the 20- and 30-ton container. Every port that functioned prior to 1945 had been built to transfer cargo in small units from seaborne to landborne carriage. Dock sheds, cranes, barges, rail wagons, and lorries were designed for loose packages. General cargo vessels were similarly constructed; staff and labour were recruited to cope with the cumbersome documentary system and to struggle to move millions of packages to and from the port or from one part of the dock to another.

In the 1950s, when the container idea was revived (in their primitive form they had been in use before 1914) and immediately expanded, the national reaction by port authorities was to accept the challenge of cargo in large boxes. They brought out the conventional heavy lifting facilities with which the port was provided. This was to ignore the first law of mechanization.[1] Continuance in this policy would have started by stifling the new traffic and ended by getting the port out of business. In the conversion of the port from its traditional job of handling small packages to that of negotiating the largest practicable cargo unit, lay problems that have by no means been finally settled. It is the re-designing of the processes that lie each side of the relatively simple job of discharging and loading containers, of which we shall treat in this and the following chapter. The study of the new container traffic involves many aspects that affect, without properly coming within, the dock estate; the least possible space will be given to these. It is only by facing up to the problems that beset them that ports will be able to survive during the next decade, and this is increasingly being recognized. Transportation in its many forms, and

[1] See p. 87.

136

most certainly on the port and shipping side, is very much the prisoner of the past. The nature of the traffic demands that all change must be evolutionary. Sugar carried in bulk as early as 1949 had to wait until it had been shown, at some considerable cost, that general-cargo space was not suitable and that special carriers were more economic. Profiting from this experience, shipowners wasted little time in attempting to wed the new traffic in containers to the centuries-old general-cargo carrier; nor were they tied down by the conventional shedding of export cargo in well-built premises. In the last few years an explosive urge has been directed to packing loose cargo into containers. Heavy financial risks must be and are being taken by ports everywhere to avoid being left behind.

Outputs and Forecasts

It was inevitable that docks built to cope with cargoes of 150 years ago have had to be closed in face of the container challenge, and this is a process that will continue. How could it be otherwise when it is predicted that 50 per cent of the world's general cargo will in the early 1980s be carried in containers?

At the major port of Rotterdam 8000 tons of cargo in containers can be discharged and loaded in 24 hours; at Tilbury in the Port of London up to forty containers have been handled in 1 hour—a rate some sixteen times greater than the normal tons-per-gang hour (Fig. 23). The container berth of today, the pride of the port, may well be the normal berth within a decade (Fig. 24). By 1970 it is confidently predicted that 300 container vessels will be in use. In 1968 there were, in the United Kingdom alone, some twenty-six ports with facilities either in use or that could be developed for handling containers (Fig. 25). On each container berth 1 million tons of cargo, it is estimated, could be handled each year.[1] There are plans for traffic between Britain and New Zealand ports, by 1972, for a fleet of ships that will each carry 1100 refrigerated containers as well of 300 containers for general cargo. The developing traffic between the ports of the United Kingdom and the Continent has disproved the earlier belief that container ships could operate successfully only on a long voyage. Despite the continued progress in the design of container ships, which has included better methods of loading and discharging, the problems inherent in the trade to the Far East have not yet been solved. The search

[1] The figure of 1 million tons of general cargo handled yearly was the lower limit of what was technically known as a "small port".

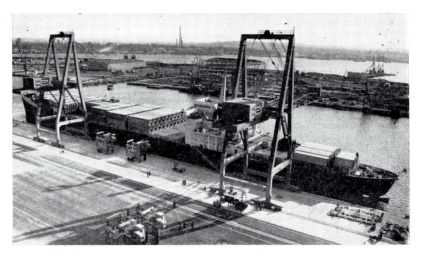

FIG. 23. The *American Lancer* from New York discharging containers at
40-berth Tilbury Dock, London. (By courtesy of PLA.)

for a solution here may concentrate on the unit load, and this may be a
mixture of containers, flats, and pallets with ships equipped with side-
loading transporters and triple hatches. No one who has watched a large
general-cargo ship taking in cargoes from lighters in Hong Kong harbour
will minimize the difficulties. Whilst the New Zealand traffic offers exceptional opportunities for the container, the fact remains that there will still
be responsibility for the cargo that cannot be packed into containers, and
this will be recognized by the shipping companies.

   In Antwerp, during the first 9 months of 1968, nearly half a million
tons of cargo in 43,000 containers was shipped; an increase of 36 per cent
over the corresponding figure for 1967.

   The figures quoted are sufficient to show how output has been revolutionized;[1] also that we are in for an era of intense competition between
ports to secure a container traffic that has by no means settled into a
final and definite pattern. One of the many problems that will have to be
faced is the congestion on the roads leading to the ports. Inadequate as
many of these now are for export traffic spread over a week's loading,

[1] Port labour costs for moving a container can be as low as one-twentieth of the cost
for the same weight of conventional cargo.

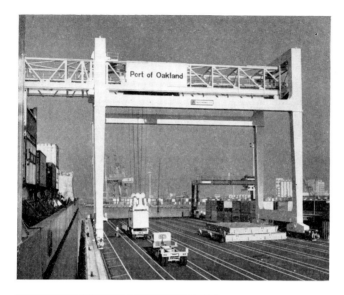

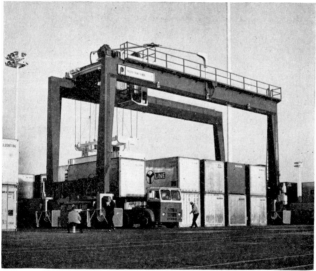

FIG. 24. Container berth at the port of Oakland, California, with PACECO
cranes. Portainer crane (*top*) and Transtainer crane (*bottom*).
(By courtesy of Paceco, Alameda, California.)

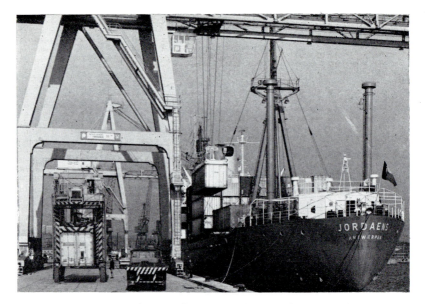

Fig. 25. Loading containers at Southampton for New York.
(By courtesy of the British Transport Dock Board.)

they will be gravely so if this tonnage is to be concentrated into a matter
of hours, and will arrive in mammoth-sized loads.

Larger Container Ships

Ships built for the container trade are already in the region of 25,000
d.w.t.[1] This is a size that would be unacceptable for general-cargo ships
because of the time taken by the first bills of lading to be loaded before
they could be discharged. Even on a mechanized berth, the clutter of
loose packages for a vessel of this size would be formidable. In the compact and more quickly handled form of containers, 25,000 d.w.t. is a
practicable figure. Now the suggestion has been made that within a few
years container ships will be treading the same path as bulk-cargo ships,
although a limit of 75,000 d.w.t. has been fixed. Never before has it been
proposed to transport general cargo, even in containers, in one ship of

[1] The *Australian Endeavour*, 24,000-ton container ship, capacity 1233 20-foot containers, left Rotterdam for Australian ports in August 1969.

this tonnage. The several problems that would be thrown up by this change will be examined later.

Advantages of Containers

Progress during the last decade has been so pronounced that it is now possible to point to material advantages that the container has brought. Firstly, it is necessary to go back to the relation between the shipper and his customer, because on the success of this will depend the smoothness with which the container traffic will flow through the port. If the size of the business permits door-to-door traffic, then the major advantages can be enjoyed. If the customer's requirement does not fill a container then, obviously, it will be a piecemeal arrangement that will involve extra costs. It is very likely that he will not desire to have his whole season's new stock delivered to him as a full container load. He may not have the money to pay for it or to get it out of bond, nor the storage space to hold it.[1] He will not want to see much of it deteriorate because his retail customers will not oblige by taking—and paying for—ten times as much as they at present need. Importers of wine are allowed in the United Kingdom, on payment of the appropriate duty, to draw from the cask the number of gallons required to execute a bottling order. It is doubtful if the national Customs would make concessions to cover part goods drawn from containers, particularly as it would not be practicable to find bonded storage for the large number of containers involved. The importer may also be aware of the danger of hazarding all his stock in one bottom, and will prefer to spread his imports over several ships. The Suez Canal is a grim reminder of vessels on which cargo has been held up (at the time of writing) for more than 3 years. Port authorities would be pleased if commercial problems were as simple as the literature advertising door-to-door container traffic suggest.

One will naturally expect, as a return for the very high capital investment (not only on the part of the port authority), a considerable reduction in freight charges as a result of the quicker turnround on which the container ship can rely. Research carried out so far indicates a saving on door-to-door costs of as much as 60 per cent on relatively simple routes such as the North Atlantic–United Kingdom, or at a figure of 40 per cent for the more complex voyages and where some inland

---

[1] A 20-foot container loaded with golf balls would be valued at £33,000, but it would certainly be far more than the importer would want in one shipment.

handling is involved. There is a different figure for each route, and the nearer the traffic approaches a simple port-to-port shuttle service, the greater the savings that will be possible. In many instances the transport company admits to having for the first time complete control of the handling from door to door. There are already signs of a freight war to secure the available traffic in containers. It may be some time before conditions will have settled down to those enjoyed in pre-container days by the major liner conferences. Neither is it to be expected that containers can be used to their full advantage in the developing countries, where the volume of traffic is insufficient for a regular service, whatever their ideas may at present be.

Economies in Manning

The few men needed to work a container ship and the phenomenal outputs achieved have been given publicity in the Press. Pensions and severance pay have been introduced to soften the blow of inevitable redundancy. A labour force from which the older and less-fit men have been weeded will in time take over the working of container ships, which will spend only $12\frac{1}{2}$ per cent of their working lives in port compared with some 56 per cent by general-cargo ships at present. Three early working records at Tilbury Dock will show how completely new ideas have taken over.

American Lynx berthed at 15.56 hours on 24 December 1968. It is a port custom that work ceases at 12.00 hours on Christmas Eve. This ship, had she had general-cargo, would have waited on the berth until making a half-hearted start after the Christmas holidays. On this occasion, however, the ship broke bulk immediately and sailed at 03.02 hours on 25 December having used only fifteen men on the ship and quay. No previous instance of a ship breaking bulk on the afternoon of Christmas Eve, in London, could be quoted.

American Legion, discharged and loaded 6600 tons in $10\frac{1}{2}$ hours. The turnround would, under general cargo conditions, have taken 200 men a week.

American Lancer arrived and broke bulk on a Bank Holiday. Because of torrential rain, work had to cease for a time because the crane driver could not see his load. The fact was demonstrated that containers can be almost 100 per cent independent of weather.

Pilferage

The onset of the container was hailed as a final solution to the grave scandal of pilferage in the docks. Organized gangs, it is true, had a set-back, and petty pilferage was driven off the market. Attention has already been paid to the problem of effectively sealing each container. It was early realized that a container may be loaded and consigned from the other side of the world and that the contents are not checked until the final destination is reached. Supervision of the sealing and the unsealing is also essential, as is the close check on the seals wherever this is possible during the journey.

Condensation has also been responsible for the introduction of a "breathing" valve which equalizes the atmospheric pressure inside the container and contains also a dessicant which dries the air passing through the valve. Problems of taint have also arisen which indicate that there is still much to learn on the internal stowage of containers.

The Role of the Port Authority

This has been briefly expressed by one port director, to create the facilities in advance of the demand—a doctrine in accordance with modern thinking. As the body responsible for administering the port, the users look to it to plan developments so that the facilities they may require will be in the right place at the right time. This is the insoluble problem with which all port authorities are faced. Where they act as operating companies for the discharge and loading of container ships, the problem is eased because they can allocate berth space very much on the lines of general-cargo berths, although the usage is at a much accelerated rate. It has, however, been found possible to give accommodation on the berth to several small container lines[1] as each company may need the berth for a few hours only, because work proceeds throughout the 24 hours of each day. Larger users have been able to reach agreement among themselves for allocation to a berth. Because of the high cost of berth equipment, cranes, forklift trucks, and straddle carriers, the port authority must do its best to ensure maximum use. A container-lifting gantry-type crane may cost up to £220,000, and no effort is wasted that will help to give it continuous use.[2] At most container ports a 24-hour mobile repair service has been instituted

---

[1] There is a common-user container berth at Tilbury Dock, London.

[2] At Bristol, two 30-ton gantry cranes operate in parallel with a common overlap area. This is known as the "Fast Random Access Method" (FRAM).

for the repair and maintenance of damaged containers as well as for essential handling equipment.

Attention has already been drawn to the difficulties in maintaining direct delivery of general cargo to rail,[1] and this has, so far, proved generally impracticable for containers. Once again it is essential that the port authority should have overall control of the berth so that the road and rail access—and this will include the depots for liner trains—comes under their control. To cut out delays, the towage service between the dock entrance and the berth, if it is an enclosed dock, will need to be looked at. It may be beneficial for the port authority to settle on an annual schedule with the shipping companies making use of the berth.

Impact on Shippers

Now that the time has passed when the more obvious advantages to shippers of containers have been accepted, attention has been, and continues to be, paid to problems such as the supply of cargo in containers to the container ships. It has been realized that only where the two-way flow of cargo is sufficient and smooth will the container service function as it should. The importance of marketing teams sent out by the shipping consortia to remove some of the difficulties the shipper will experience between the factory and the dock, has been accepted. Their work has been summed up —to see that the containers fit the loading bays and will go through the factory gates.[2] This will include a large range of problems that have not before arisen because the conventional traffic has been built up on lines to suit the manually handled package. The container will certainly develop as an acceptable piece of handling equipment in industries that are not big enough to support their container services on their own.[3] In this process, the shipping and forwarding agent has an important part to play, more important than his traditional role of midwife to the conventional package cargo bill of lading. While it will not be difficult for the agent to take responsibility for the full container load and to treat it very much as a normal large package, there are problems of the "less than container load" where his expertise will prove valuable. He will arrange

---

[1] See p. 134.

[2] Mr. A. J. Macintosh, Commercial Manager, Associated Container Transportation.

[3] Container ships as "transport vehicles" are now possible. They are for short and intermediate sea trade, they are small (1700 tons), and can be leased on bareboat charter. Ten of these ships are contemplated.

to concentrate these small parcels where they can be "grouped" or "consolidated" with other cargo, with which they can travel, into a full container load. His knowledge of conditions will enable him to choose the most appropriate service and the most economical route for the goods. He could, if he has a liking for the jargon of the computer age, describe himself as a consultant. By working together, forwarding agents who will not have control of traffic sufficient in size to fill their own containers, expect to be able to ensure regular services of containers filled with compatible cargo. The influence that a trusted forwarding agent can exert on his principal—the shipper—to vary his packaging methods so that they will the more easily fit the stowing of containers, will be important.

The two-way flow of containers is the justification for the existence of marketing teams. They naturally seek perfection, but they are conscious that shipping is the one industry where it is not attainable. For years to come the problem of returning empty containers will have to be faced, probably until universal container pools operate. There will always be markets where the flow of cargo in the opposite direction is not suitable, or, in fact, may not exist. Here advantage can be taken of "folding" containers, the return freight on which is a quarter only of that of the full container.

Impact on Importers

The best understanding of the part that the national Customs are playing in their assessment of container traffic can be gained by looking at the problem through the eyes of a practical Customs landing officer. Used to having cargo produced to him so that he can see the contents, can even probe bales of wool or hemp for concealed contraband, he is now faced with a large box of some 15–25 tons of mixed goods. Chances of concealment and misrepresentation are possible because of the greater difficulties of access to certain parcels. At the same time, the high cost of delay brings pressure on the Customs for greater speed in clearance. They welcome the greater security against pilferage that the container normally provides, the likelihood of better documentation, and the possibility of introducing automatic data-processing techniques to do away with routine controls.

In the past, Customs drill has been concentrated on the ports where, as the first place of entry, goods dutiable and non-dutiable can be canalized across the quays either at the dock of discharge or at the wharf where the barge, under Customs lock, will discharge. Sealed containers have now made possible the secure transit of general cargo in bulk form, and national Customs are now prepared to clear goods in containers at recognized inland depots (Fig. 26). In France Customs officers will clear parcels at importers' premises.

It remains, and national Customs are right in emphasizing this point, that speed of clearance depends on the proper action being taken by the importer—either himself or through an agent. Someone must tell the guardians of the revenue what is being imported; if need be, a plan of the interior packing of the container—a miniature ships' plan in fact—can

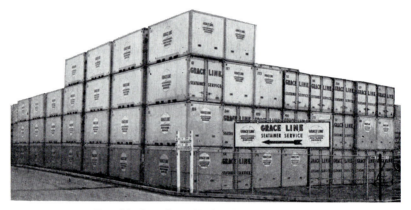

FIG. 26. Containers filled and waiting disposal.

be produced to aid in locating a particular parcel. It will be essential that a means of communication is used that will make certain that entries can be presented before the arrival of the container. In many instances—and it should be borne in mind that Customs officers have become, with their unrivalled experience of goods and human nature, highly selective and time saving in what they choose to examine—it will be possible for the container just landed, or just arrived at the depot, to be loaded and removed without going through the Customs' control. Breaking-down at a depot of "less than container load" consignments has been a help to the Customs since the inception of container traffic. The Customs on their part have been generally helpful in devising means of avoiding delays and in con- sulting the various interested parties. This is particularly the case with the problem of containers that are imported empty for future use. The variety of operations that the working of international container pools promise will call for this measure of co-operation with national Customs.

Tallying, that most unproductive of dock processes, has in its present form, no future with containers. In fact the growing tonnage of cargo carried in containers is directly robbing the tally clerk of his traditional work; it is also making an appreciable saving in terminal costs. Under the plans made for major United Kingdom container ports, a completely computer-controlled cargo-handling system will take over the movement of containerized cargo from the port of origin to the destination. The computer system will comprise seven interlinked systems: import and exports; transport control and container control; freight accounting and financial accounting; and also management information. There is no place in such a system for a man sheltering from the rain making marks on a card.

When air companies entered the freight market they sensibly cut documentation down to the bone. The traditional system of documenting general cargo has produced a clutter of paper added to by each separate interest that takes its turn in passing, or helping to pass, the bill of lading on its journey and assumes, for a limited time, responsibility for the cargo. What a deterrent it is to the British export market to have to cope with conditions where a consignment, after taking perhaps 3 months from factory to destination, arrives partly damaged with little chance for the consignee to disentangle the paper chains that prevent his pinning down the guilty party. How attractive it must seem to an importer to get his goods from a supplier in a neighbouring country where only a frontier barrier has to be raised. Computer control of a major container berth will help to produce a system where the arrival of each container will be known and anticipated, its position on the berth determined, and its stowage in the ship recorded. Traditional movements of cargo within the berth has relied for its successful working on good supervision with the human element predominating. Errors cost money. If the claims made that computers do not make mistakes are substantiated, the role of the supervisory staff as we have always understood it will be in for a very drastic revision.

Standardization of Container Sizes

In the 1950s, when it was realized that containers had come to stay, the advantages of a standard-size container were apparent. There were other aspects, mostly operational, where benefit to all handlers of containers were equally apparent. In 1961 the International Standards Organization set up a committee, ISO/TC/104, to make recommendations for the standardization of containers having an external volume of 1 m³ (35·3 ft³) or greater, as regards terminology, classification, dimensions, specifications, test methods, and marking. Three working groups to cover these separate fields began their work in that year, and in 1964 the committee produced its final recommendations on dimensions and ratings. In the following year the committee considered questions of specifications, testing, and the marking of freight containers. Attention was also paid to the important points involved in corner fittings, for it was accepted that standardized equipment for lifting containers would depend on standardized fitments and that time would be saved in each container crane cycle if attachment of the container to the spreader was automatic.

Large containers very properly came in for the early work of the committee, and agreement was reached on two simple categories. Series 1, designated 1A to 1F containers, all 8 ft high and 8 ft wide but having lengths from 40 ft down to as low as 5 ft. Their capacity ranged from 30 tons for containers 1A to 5 tons for 1F. Series 2 covered three types of containers, 2A, 2B, and 2C with a constant capacity of 7 tons but with varying dimensions. Several matters that were pertinent to operating requirements were also dealt with. A difficulty with which the committee had to contend was that the design of containers was not, and never would be, stationary. Therefore many design modifications were considered in the knowledge that an optional requirement (to quote an authority on container standardization and a member of ISO/TC/104)[1] "demanded by users generally, is likely in due course to be made obligatory; one which only a few users want may eventually lose its optional status".[2]

The consideration of the external size of the large containers led to the knotty problem of how best to make use of the valuable internal space. How to employ pallets which had already had international sizes conferred on them by the United Nations a few years earlier. Modulation is the key to the effective use of space whether for unit loads, pallets, or

[1] Mr. E. S. Tooth, MBE, lately Docks Manager, Port of London Authority, India and Millwall Docks, London.
[2] The sizes standardized have not, however, met with universal approval, and recent additions to container fleets show that there is, in some countries, a strong movement towards increasing the height of containers to 8 ft 6 in, or even 9 ft.

loose packages. If the modular problems of pallets and containers can be solved, then the container floors must be strong enough to stand the weight of loaded forklift trucks. Similarly, weatherproof testing is necessary because containers are stowed on the deck of the carrying ship, and it is the exception to give loaded containers shed space whilst they are on the berth or at the depot. This led to the consideration of the major equipment used in moving containers in these and other places.

Finally, agreement was reached in June 1968 on a number of matters the most serious of which were corner fittings. What to a layman would seem to be a very minor matter, whether the fitments should be recessed or should protrude, would mean a saving of hold space in the first case as against a serious loss if the alternative was forced. All port operators are aware that to every agreed principle there is an exception; despite direful prophecies the exception somehow works. So it was with containers. Despite the hard work that the committee put in, some enterprises that had already devised their own form of container are big enough to adhere to this and to ignore the recommendations of ISO/TC/104.

Sympathy must go to the committee for the impossible job that the International Standards Organization set them. The size of the container was originally influenced by the size of road and rail vehicles, by the width of national roads, by the dimensions of bridges and tunnels—particularly the latter. Weight-bearing capacity of the carrier also played its part. In the United States these are generally larger than the standards accepted for European countries. With the desperate need to reduce costs and to overcome restrictive port practices, the Americans can hardly be expected to adopt a container that is smaller than those which they know full well can daily be employed internally. The ISO container is an international one; to separate those which can from those which cannot continue their journey on shipboard would be an intolerable handicap to the American shipper.

In the early months of 1969 the Inland Transport Committee of the Economic Commission for Europe noted a growing tendency to build containers which did not conform to ISO standards, and they have set themselves to obtain (July 1969) information on the extent to which "non-standard" containers, differing in height, width, and length, or in handling fixtures from types recommended by ISO are being built or envisaged. They also propose to exploit the extent to which at ports operational and technical difficulties might arise from the use of containers which deviate from international standards. There are also safety aspects of using containers exceeding the height and width recommended by ISO, particularly in connection with the routing of such containers by road or rail. They would also wish to cover the purposes to be served and the economic advantages to be derived from the use of non-standard containers.

At the time of writing the position would seem to be that an international-type container has been agreed and recommended. It is likely that it will be used in what might be described as "permanent" container traffic routes where shipping consortia have effective control of the transportation; this will cover much of the business emanating from European ports as well as from the United Kingdom. At the same time the non-conforming movement, limited probably to specialized trades, is of sufficient size to call for investigation by a body of the status of the Economic Commission for Europe. Just as standardization in the construction of freight-carrying ships has always been beaten by the shipowner's particular requirements, so shippers who are big enough to apply this principle to containers will continue to do so to their own advantage.

Additional Notes

Chapter 9, page 140, footnote 1. Ship building programme. OCL are (July 1970) building five ships of 38,000 d.w.t. for the Pacific trade. Containers will be stacked nine high under deck with ten rows athwart ship.

Page 149, par. 1. Half containers are now made for ingots with specially strengthened floors.

CHAPTER 10

THE CONTAINER TRAFFIC II

The Container Ship

Mention has already been made[1] of the attempts to handle the early types of containers as heavy lifts. Like so many innovations in cargo handling, containers took some time to develop away from the general-cargo ship. An early type of ship, which was in effect a bulk carrier, took forty-two containers. This was succeeded by the larger and cellular type with capacities from 200 to over 600 20-ton containers. Orders were placed in December 1968 for ships that would carry 1500 standard 20-ton containers each.

But there are conditions in which it is economic to load general cargo alongside containers, and this principle has been carefully worked out in a fleet of six container ships, the first of which sailed from London in June 1969. The total cargo capacity of each ship will be 1 million ft^3 of which 192,000 ft^3 is for cargo not in containers, and 275,000 ft^3 for refrigerated consignments. It is likely that this combined cargo will persist subject to more and more of the present loose cargo being carried ultimately in the ship's cellular space. It is unlikely that new vessels of any size will be designed and built exclusively for the deep-sea break-bulk trades.

Some of the early containers were carried on wheels in the well-deck of a roll-on vessel. This was an operation so simple to perform—the loading and the discharge were in fact done by the lorry driver—that little time elapsed before the principle of the combined roll-on and container ship found expression in new building for the Europe–North America traffic. The loss of cargo space in the carrying holds is set off by the greater flexibility. With these dual-purpose vessels the shipping company is in the market for finished cars from Sweden to Canada. It is a far cry from

[1] See p. 136.

151

the making of false decks and enclosing cars in skeleton metal frames to protect them during handling of a decade ago. Where small containers are stowed in general hold space, it is anticipated that these will be capable of being moved around by one man on a "hoverpallet", an application of the air-cushion principle.

Attention has been given for cross-channel services, to catamaran vessels, envisaged as being 240 ft long and 68 ft wide, each carrying 110 containers; these would be stowed mainly on the deck linking the two hulls. If the project should take shape between London and a major French port, it would revolutionize the cross-channel cargo services.

For overseas traffic container ships are now being planned with speeds of 25–30 knots. For the first time in the history of shipping, speed on the ocean will be matched by speed on turnround. Expensive improvements to add a few knots to speed will no longer be negatived by exasperating delays in port.

The last word has not been spoken on the handling gear suitable for containers. Despite the heavy weight of deck gantry gear and the subtraction that this makes to the carrying capacity of the ship, the claim is made that by having the gear literally spread over the deck of the ship and giving access to all the cells, much time is saved and more containers can be handled than with the quay crane. The controversy between the usefulness of ships' gear and quay cranes looks like being extended to container ships.

The Container Berth

Loading expensively built containers into a still more expensively built ship is a far cry from the native labour that humped a few bales of tobacco into the hold of a sailing ship. It was not very material how long so small an investment remained on the primitive berth that in those far-off days made possible the transfer from land to water-borne transport. So great is the investment in the container berth, commencing with the vast area of the quay, perhaps as much as 20 acres, and also the background space, through the valuable gear with which the cargo is handled, right into the cellular ship that cost several million pounds to build, that an entirely new approach from the traditional is now needed (Fig. 27). If a berth of some 1000 ft long could be used intensively, then ten times the throughput of a general cargo berth could be handled. Obviously the highly specialized facilities of a container berth must be extensively exploited.[1] By preventing the irresponsible spreading of container berths the port authority will be able to ensure the most intense and the most economical use of the few they have.

It will mean that a phenomenal tonnage will be pinpointed on one relatively small part of the port, but it is very much to the point that staff

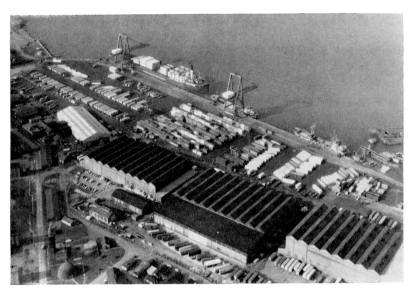

FIG. 27. Felixstowe container harbour—aerial view.
(By courtesy of Felixstowe Dock and Railway Co.)

such as dockmasters, engineers, executive, and supervisory staff concerned with the berth should be kept as fully occupied as possible. If, however, a greater depth of water should be needed, it will be convenient for this to be localized to one part of the dock. The width of entrance locks may have to be revised. A single lock might mean restricted working, and this would

---

[1] From *The Port*, 25 September 1969: "Record shipments were made from Tilbury's multi-user (container) berth No. 43 in the second week in September. Over 1200 containers were handled—100 more than the previous figure. Main users of the berth are European Unit Routes who run daily to Rotterdam and thrice weekly to Antwerp and also Dunkirk. The United Baltic Corporation, Finland Steamship Company and Oy Finlines Limited, also use the berth for their container service about every five days to Helsinki. The East German Line run a weekly container service to Rostock."

be a temptation to open up a berth down river outside the impounded area with a consequent loss of dues to the authority.

There is no standard size decreed for the berth. Ships range around 700 ft in length with an actual working run less than this. Provision for loading and discharging some 1200 containers has to be made. Access by road and rail is important; there should normally be room at either end of the ship for shipping off containers by barge.

An alternative to the horizontal short-term housing of containers has been suggested in a container park. This embodies the principle of a multistorey car park. Starting from the assumption that 2000 20-foot containers could be parked in one installation, it is claimed that this would take up about 1 acre instead of the 20 or more that ports like Amsterdam are providing. The following operations (among others) are claimed for the equipment included: the container can be placed, from its position on the quay, into the storage tower—a twin elevator within the tower does this; Customs requirements can easily be met; a container can be removed from the tower within 90 seconds and automatically loaded on to road or rail transport. All operations affecting the receipt, movement, and dispatch of cargo are recorded by computers: all containers are put under cover which, with temperature and humidity changes, could be a very valuable asset in other than temperate countries. Lastly, there is concentration rather than a controlled sprawl. In smaller ports where land is not available for expansion, an installation of this kind would be valuable.

In the many descriptions that have appeared of container berths throughout the world, very little has been written of the superb organization that must be produced in a single effort by shipping companies, forwarding agents, rail, and road interests if the turnover of 25–30 containers an hour is to be kept up. Like many other processes in cargo handling, attention is apt to be directed to the physical operation of taking cargo out of the ship and putting other cargo in. Without the meticulous care that produces the container ready to load and can arrange for another container to be delivered, the spectacular process of handling 30-ton containers would soon come to a halt. It could be fortunate that the arrival of containers coincided with that of computers.

An encouraging feature of the part played by rail in the new container traffic has been, in the United Kingdom, the alacrity with which British Rail has accepted the challenge. They have seen their job as providing direct service between the major ports and selected inland centres. Their boast has been "next morning" deliveries; recently some 5000 cases of imported apples were loaded on open-sided freight liner containers in the Port of London and were being sold in Glasgow the next day. In such journeys as these the railways have the obvious edge over road transport and this will make competition more keen.

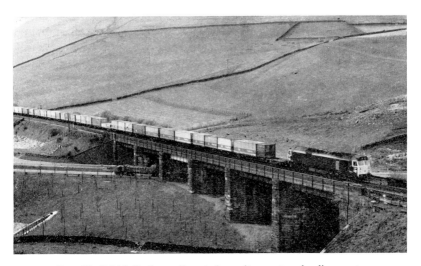

Fig. 28. British Railways liner train on its way to a loading port.
(By courtesy of British Railways Board.)

Freight trains are made up with three large-sized containers on each rail wagon; they are loaded by transverse gantries, and there are special wagons for traffic that calls for non-standard sized containers (Fig. 28). Needless to say, the transport of containers in this manner was very quickly taken up by the cross-Channel rail ferry services. Every week a liner service links up, as between Antwerp and Rotterdam, at Cologne and travels non-stop to Milan.

Already there have been some adjustments in the continental rail-handling methods. Many ports operators consider that containers can be better handled if removed directly from the berth to an assembly area in the rear, there to be made up into freight liner trains. Once more the dubious value of direct ship-to-rail traffic obtrudes. At Tilbury Dock a reorganization of the rail-handling arrangements has put two shifts a day to work the trains in the terminal and to and from the container berth.

That height counts for more in handling cargo than area was the major discovery of the age of mechanization. It would be strange if it had not been almost immediately applied to containers. We have referred already to the container park. There is no doubt that the piling of containers either as a separate stack or performed by the crane that does the loading and discharge of the ship, will encroach on earlier ideas of horizontal storage with unlimited room. In this system the transversing gantry has a sweep of 180 ft on which it can place containers three high, and for a length determined by the crane rails inset on the quay. Thus a high proportion, if not all the cargo at any one time, may be on the quay and under plumb.

Mechanical Requirements for Berth

In 1959 the first port-based gantry container crane was erected at Alameda in California. This was most thoroughly thought out and set the pattern for later developments. The gantry crane and its lifting apparatus must be able to place a container into any ship cell. It must also be able to load and unload highway trailers on the quay. It has the advantage over the ship's transverse gantry in that it has a constant plumb unaffected by the list that the ship may take as the load swings across to the wings. It must be said in favour of ships' gear that the ship is independent of shore-based equipment and that this makes for flexibility. Also it opened up the far side, or overside, so that containers could be lifted direct from craft.

The shore-based crane, in common with the ship crane, will unload the container directly on to the road vehicle at the ship's side. It will remain on this while parked on the berth, during its journey to its destination, and until ready for outward loading. Against the advantages of a single handling must be set the tying up of the vehicle; there must be a chassis for every container ashore. The alternative "ground storage" system provides for the container to be placed on to a transferring vehicle at the ship's side, or it may be put down directly on the quay. A truck will move the container from its position under plumb on to the space allotted to it in the storage area. As containers can be piled three high less storage ground is required and trailers are not kept under load; shore cranes of the future will probably have a span in width up to 150 ft so as to provide room for storage and the stacking of containers under the base of the crane, and this will provide a reserve for loading when the process starts. It will also reduce the amount of operating ground required and the number of transfers that have to be made. It will be an important development because it is a direct contribution to improving the crane cycle and hence the tonnage handled per hour. A further point is that shore cranes are now being built with increased height under the boom so as to allow higher deck loading, particularly on ships with a high freeboard.

The general "hardware" of the berth has, in the last decade, produced a variety of efficient heavy-duty machinery. There are certain basic jobs to be done, starting with the arrival of freight liner trains, their unloading, and the transfer of the containers to storage positions. This may involve the use of forklift trucks, including side loaders, swing lift, and double-stacking and carrying vehicles[1] as well as specially designed lifting devices, some of which can pile containers three high. Provision has similarly to be made for large arrivals by road and rail. An interesting development was the adaptation of the spreader so that there should be no delay in clamping this on to the container whilst at the same time it damped out all movement of the load by a high wind. This would have been sufficient to delay the placing of the container in its appropriate cell by several seconds. There are now self-levelling spreaders which are worked by a sensing device; also a telescopically adjusted spreader that can be adapted to various lengths of containers up to 40 ft.

Design and Types of Containers

Whilst attention has been directed to the problems of standardizing, not only the containers but the equipment with which they have been handled, a great deal of work has been put in on devising containers for special commodities. Gradually the number of items that can be packed into containers increases. Not only has ingenuity been shown in packing a conventional item such as wool into containers—shipped as loose bales for more than 100 years—but for special commodities containers have now been adapted or re-designed. The early bulk-liquid transport container, with a stainless-steel lining, holding 585 gallons and weighing only 2 tons, has given way to the 24,000-gallon stainless-steel tank that carries wine from Australia with no loss from evaporation or taint to the contents.

---

[1] There is now a straddle carrier that will lift two containers, carry and stack both, and has a lifting capacity of 70,000 lb.

Smaller tanks will carry 8400 gallons and some have three compartments (each holding 2000 gallons) for different kinds of wine.

Refrigerated containers have always appealed to the shipper of frozen and chilled meat. They see in insulating a small cubic capacity an economy against having to do this for a complete hold, even when there is only a small quantity of cargo to be carried. Chilled beef is now being brought from Poland. Frozen beef that is transported at $0°F$ and vegetables that require only a cool temperature of $34-38°F$, can be carried in refrigerated containers that are divided into two compartments. There is much scope for bacon and butter from Denmark, and this has now been organized on a door-to-door system. Carbon black, that most objectionable and penetrating of cargoes, has been carried in special containers, but for those consignees who still want their shipments in bags, a large unit load of these has been placed inside a double prefabricated cardboard container which makes the load safe against any possible spillage. A similar contrivance is a plastic-coated collapsible fabric sack container which will carry $1\frac{1}{2}$ tons and can, it is claimed, be used for more than 100 journeys. It has a steel collar for lifting by crane or derrick, and a stable base; it is ideal for exporting dry raw materials.

"Flats" are a species of container with a solid base and a headpiece; they can be fitted, as to the remaining three sides, with weld mesh, and are ideal for loose ironmongery, unpacked sanitary ware, or machine tools. Open-top containers through which coke, coal, grain, ore, or scrap metal can be loaded, are fitted with a hinged-end door. They have strong floors that will take a loaded forklift truck if it is desired to fill them with unit loads. Some types have vertically hinged centre opening doors or sides that will collapse to allow long members to be loaded with side-lifting forklift trucks. It was early realized that standard-sized containers are not really suitable for heavy cargo, i.e. that which is 40 ft^3 or less to the ton. Few parcels are more laborious to handle than ingots of metal, slabs of copper, or bundles of tin plates. For such high-density cargo the half-height container has been invented where the height is 4 ft instead of 8. Sides and ends are built of steel framing with strong plywood panels, and the side frames can be removed for ease in loading. An all-welded steel underframe gives the strength needed for such heavy cargo and prevents the framework from twisting and warping when in use.

In the urge to find the larger cargo unit there is endless scope for the type and variety of container that can be used in moving cargo.

The Terminal Depot

Although it is unlikely to be found in the port area—and there are good reasons why this should be so—the terminal depot cannot be dissociated from the berth. In the United States there would not seem to have been very much opposition by dockworkers to the process of "stuffing" being done by outside labour, i.e. the job of stowing small parcels of less than container load. In the United Kingdom, shipping lines have had their hands forced by a custom of the port that ordains that dockers handle loose exports in the stages prior to shipment. This has been held to confer on the dockers the right to do this work, although both in London and Liverpool the depots are some miles away from the docks. The depots will throughout their operation be manned by dockers; this will give employment to some of the many elderly dockers who are now redundant. The main interest that port authorities will have (and the number of terminal depots will certainly increase) is that the work should be done in an efficient way and that there is no delay in feeding exports to the berth or in dealing with the contents of containers removed from the berth. During the arguments over the manning of depots it was advanced that women would be capable of doing the work, that piecework as known in the docks would be unsuitable, and that shift and weekend working would be necessary. Against this it was put forward that only dockers have the expert knowledge of cargo behaviour and the niceties of stowage. In addition, and this no doubt swayed the decision, there is redundancy, everywhere brought about by the container; there are older and less able dockers for whom work has to be found.

On the siting of the depots it is necessary to obtain the co-operation of the national Customs who must be satisfied that there will be no less to the revenue through their examination of dutiable cargo at a point remote from that of first importation.

As to the actual stowing of consignments of less than container load, there is little to be said. Swedish shippers have, through ICHCA, already worked on problems of standardization, and there is little doubt that the work will fall into well-recognized practices. There are certainly matters regarding strains that arise in loading and unloading, setting cargo at safety inside flats and containers, and also humidity and condensation. There is also room at the terminal depot for experiment with air pillows as dunnage and similar contrivances that will ensure safe arrival of delicate contents. It is reasonable to expect that considerable expertise will develop in selecting like parcels for stowage in the same container. Such exports as fragile vacuum flasks will invite modular packaging so as to produce a tight load in the standard container. There should be some variety in the containers waiting to be stowed so that all kinds of cargo from light electronics to heavy-density metals can find appropriate and homogeneous stowage.

Finally, the damage sustained by the improperly stowed contents of containers in the earlier stages proved that those responsible for packing them had regarded the container merely as another form of packing—which it is not. The container is the outward form taken by the unit load—one may repeat that it is in fact the ultimate form of unit load. The contents must therefore be assembled and made, by packing, into a single unit that is, preferably, based on modular packaging by exporters. Only thus can damage-free transit be guaranteed.

General

The ultimate pattern of the container traffic, which ports will assume the role of main container ports and which will settle down into subsidiary feeder ports where containers can be shipped coastwise, has not yet been settled. Until 1968 it was argued that one main port would suffice for each country, and that whole areas such as the Mediterranean and the Near East could be served by one port that was, in turn, fed from feeder ports to the growth of which no limit would be set. It has not worked out in this neat way which would, no doubt, have pleased the planners and economists but no one else. Whilst—in the United Kingdom—London, Southampton, and Liverpool were each reluctant to yield, and all asserted the physical advantages that they claimed gave them precedence, smaller ports got on with the job. The seaside resort of Felixstowe, popular with Edwardian summer visitors, has in the last few years concentrated on containers rather than concerts, and has developed a first-class business with Rotterdam, taking advantage of its nearness to that port. Harwich, which for many years maintained a tenuous passenger service with Holland, came into prominence in 1957 with its container and palletized traffic. To these it has added vehicle ferries. Grimsby, prominent as a fishing port for generations, now has its roll-on services that include the carriage of containers. Among the Forth ports, Grangemouth—always an efficient port for cargo handling—has become prominent through the volume of its new container traffic, and boasts that it was the first port to have two cranes working on the one quay. On the other side of Great Britain, containers for the Irish ports of Belfast and Dublin are being handled through Holyhead.

Enough has been said to indicate that making provision for containers is a tender subject, not always decided by economics but sometimes by politics. The ban on the traffic imposed by the dockers' unions at the new container berths at Tilbury in 1969 gave a tremendous fillip to small ports on the east coast of Great Britain that could ship containers to Rotterdam and Antwerp for loading there. In the eyes of the three major United Kingdom ports, container berths have come to be regarded too much as a status symbol; the present proliferation of berths could lead to a cut-throat competition as is already being felt in United States ports and, at the worst, bankruptcy for the unfortunate. This view, however, does not give enough weight to several real advantages that small ports enjoy; the cheap price of new frontage for berths, uncluttered road and rail approaches, and often a nearness to industrial centres. There would seem to be a field for the development of the small container vessel carrying about 100 containers. In the interests of economy a gross tonnage of some 1200 tons, a length of 230 ft, and a draft of 16 ft 6 in. is envisaged. Known generally as "coastal container ships", they would be eminently suitable for traffic in European waters. The LASH ships, with their lighters loaded with containers, are already equipped to off-load these for coastal service as well as for serving the wharves to be found on estuarial waters—perhaps some miles from the nearest seaport.

Insurance is not a subject that directly affects the efficient handling of cargo in a port. It is worth mentioning because of the difficulties, many of them not anticipated, that have come to light as the traffic has developed. To pack a large box with a number of light and vulnerable cargo units would seem to be the ideal way of minimizing damage in transit, if not—as many of the pioneers in the 1950s asserted—removing it altogether from the picture of dock and ship handling. However, the many teething troubles, not yet overcome, have gravely disappointed underwriters as well as perplexing shippers.[1] It is necessary to accept the fact that the larger cargo unit is one form of concentrating the risk. To express this simply, if a box

---

[1] The many grave accidents that can happen to containers and their contents are referred to in an article in the *ICHCA Journal* for November 1969, p. 26: "Underwriters—are they justifiably container shy?", by Captain William F. Warm.

of oranges falls off a hand truck very little harm, apart from a fractional bruising of the contents, is likely to happen. If, however, a container is dropped, every package therein is liable to be damaged, the extent and nature of which can be determined only by opening and examining all the contents—itself an expensive process. If a container were to be dropped on to other containers in stowage or on the quay, the "mess" would take quite a lot of clearing up. Whilst pilferage on the conventional small scale has become increasingly difficult, the hijacking of the complete container is not improbable. The need for expert packers has been mentioned, and the process must also take account of the differing densities of the contents and the likelihood of their shifting during the manipulation of the container. Condensation and sweating are real problems, particularly where the voyage alternates between hot and cold climates. Contents such as chocolate, tinned milk, films, etc., should not be subjected to tropical heat.

Apart from these risks there is the major problem of how to protect the contents of containers from the weather, including the notorious gales of the North Atlantic. Some 40 per cent of the traffic is carried on deck, and on some general-cargo ships they may be stowed four high. Because they have stood up to the handling on road and rail is not a guarantee that they will withstand the buffetting of a winter voyage across the Atlantic. Although the cubic space occupied is very much less, the conditions of ventilation that are standard in the hold of a modern general-cargo ship would be hard to achieve in containers carried on deck.

In an emergency the master of a cargo ship does not hesitate to jettison his deck cargo; a softwood timber ship may reach port with a portion of her deck cargo swept overboard during the voyage. It is hardly necessary to remark that the shipper of the container, or what is more likely, the several shippers of the contents of one container, does not have nor can have any say in which containers would have to be jettisoned nor those that the sea might select as its victims.

A package deal insurance has (1969) been suggested by a large consortia to cover the miscellaneous contents of a mixed container and to simplify the taking out of insurance. Instead of each shipper arranging his own, the consortia assume liability for the full value of each item and this includes the whole journey from consignor to consignee. If damage does occur, the lengthy inquiry to find out at what stage in the journey this did in fact happen, will take place only after full and prompt settlement has been made. The element of insurance will be combined with the freight charge, and it is a feature of the scheme that limitation of carriers' liability and argument over the apportionment of responsibility for damage will have no place therein. Neither will the shipper's past record for claims count. There are problems to be solved before all will run smoothly, but the package deal does recognize that the many shippers who will be interested in the safe arrival of a 30-ton container and its contents will have to be treated differently from the shipper of, say, 1000 cases of oranges or a few casks of wine.

The Container or Land Bridge

A new concept for containers, the container bridge, at present in its early stages of development, holds sufficient promise for the future because of the essentially sensible basis on which it will be built, to affect the working conditions and the turnover in many major ports. At present (1969) it is operating between the ports of northern Europe and North America. Containers are being shipped to east coast ports of Great Britain, transferred by British Rail to the port of Manchester, and reshipped to ports on the east coast of North America. Over 100 containers a week are already moving in both directions on this new route.

Progress has also been made with the alternative route to the Far East from western Europe via Russia and Siberia to Japanese ports and ports further east. As it means using railways on both sides of the Iron Curtain and also the little-known port of Nakhodka (Vladivostok, being Russia's Far Eastern military port, cannot be used for civil traffic), and as there may be political repercussions at any time, the interests who are out to expand this traffic still have much with which to contend.[1]

Mammoth Container Ships

Bound up with the shape that the port of the future will take, is the development of container traffic and, particularly, the size of the ships that will carry them. Until quite recently this was held to have a practical

---

[1] The United States Department of Commerce (August 1969) raised the question of whether further thought would not have to be given to the Europe–United States–Far East container bridge. The many chances of missed interchange, with delays to trains and ships, was stressed. A two-span arrangement where ocean-going cargoes would be transferred to a United States terminal interchange for the remaining sea-leg to the Far East, was suggested as a preferable alternative. Savings already quoted for time and costs were questioned.

limit of some 25,000 d.w.t., and for this there were considered to be excellent reasons. Ignoring the changes that have already come about, it can be said that the port of the present is the result of developments over the last 150 years—the period of the enclosed docks. Whether we realize it or not, the pattern to which we have always been used has been based on a single factor—the very simple one of gang-hour tonnage—in 1939 around 25 tons; anything above this was good. For export cargo it was naturally less, but this varied with the stowage conditions. The size of the ship matched the time taken to discharge and load, apart from other circumstances like tide and depth of water. No one wanted a ship of 50,000 d.w.t. that would take weeks to discharge, would imprison the bottom consignments of exports for several weeks, would overwhelm the dock sheds, and exhaust the supply of port's craft. Therefore the size of the quay, of the shed, the layout of the rail sidings, the size of the labour force and the supervisory staff, the number of cranes, and the capacity of the port's warehouses—all these had come to comply with the size that the ships using the ports had, over the years, dictated.[1]

The number of ships gainfully occupied in supplying the needs of consumers all over the world is determined by, among other things, the money a country can find to pay for its imports. The availability of these imports, the frequency during the year that they are wanted, and the arrangements that can be made to receive and to distribute these supplies, are very pertinent. All in all, the problems have resolved themselves over the years, and industry operates smoothly. The nice balance that has been built up depends on how many tons of a certain commodity can be absorbed each year.

It will be convenient to consider the case of a normal middle-class couple because there are millions of them. It is the pattern that their life has taken *that determines how many ships plough their way across the seven seas.* In the course of the years the wife has become very much a creature of habit. She buys very much the same quantity of staple foods for her family each week. Every week she spends approximately the same amount over the counter of the local supermarket. The food industry is familiar with her way of life and that of millions like her. The structure of

---

[1] Consider the position of a shipper with a consignment of 50 tons of steel rods if stowed on the ceiling of a 50,000 d.w.t. general-cargo ship. It would remain there for weeks whilst the ship was loading and, after the voyage, for weeks whilst the ship was being discharged. Consider the financial loss involved.

its business is built up on this. How many tons of New Zealand butter, of Indian tea, of South African citrus fruit, or of Greek dried fruits has it to store and have available for continuous distribution against her weekly demand? Bear in mind that the storage of these and other similar commodities is only possible in first-class accommodation, and that this is expensive to build and maintain. However, the annual turnover has been most carefully calculated and the system works satisfactorily. It could, with truth, be said to take account of the size of the domestic larder, the smallest room in the house.

The husband is a director of a manufacturing firm that uses a certain amount of asbestos, in bags, and this is necessary to its finished product. It needs X tons yearly. Its works have been planned to produce finished goods for a demand that stands at Y tons yearly. Storage space is at a premium and the firm's programme of imports has been worked out so as to keep reserves of asbestos at a safe minimum. Certainly the firm's output could be increased, but this would mean rebuilding.

Both Mr. and Mrs. Consumer have geared the satisfaction of their needs to the speed with which goods can be handled in the national ports. Whatever experts may say about the quicker turnround of shipping, there is no outright and general dissatisfaction with the present ways of working.

It is evident that the pattern that ports have taken has had its influence on systems of distribution and, in fact, everything to do with the storage of goods, commencing with the size of the home larder. Whether the system is right or wrong, and the deep-freeze has already scratched the surface,[1] the fact remains that a great deal of planning depends on it.

And now comes the container ship to breach the well-established system that has ruled the country for so long. At present it has a capacity slightly in excess of that of the general-cargo ship it is in process of replacing. The container cargo is discharged and a new one loaded in a matter of hours. If we were to assume that the cargo of one such container ship consisted of, as to two-thirds, of canned fruit, tea, and asbestos, this means that the receivers are faced with collecting and absorbing cargo that might previously have taken several days to discharge. Like the bulk-cargo ship, the container ship does not, as the general-cargo ship does, spend more than 50 per cent of its life in port; it can make more voyages a year and

---

[1] It will be many years before the deep-freeze replaces the present pattern of retail buying.

will be back sooner with a similar cargo. Time will show whether the importers in this and other countries can continue their present arrangements with this hotted-up rate of importation of their cargoes.

Although there is a quicker port turnround and a probable reduction in terminal costs that should follow this, demand will not suddenly shoot up overnight. The amount of sugar the housewife buys does not depend on its cost—in this case it is affected by social reasons. Due to the changeover, since 1949, from bag to bulk it has been possible to keep costs over the counter down. There is, in fact, already a world over-production of sugar. Similarly, the consumption of tinned soups would not double because they are now carried in containers which are very expeditiously handled at the docks.

If the size of container ships remained as at present, one can visualize supply and demand, after a violent see-saw in the early stages, settling down as the same quantity, more or less, found its way into the country in containers instead of cartons. The effect of interfering with the accepted method of shipping a staple product was illustrated in the turnover from the whole fruit to the juice only, of oranges from Florida to New York. The quantity of juice that the ship could carry in her tanks was found to be greater than the market could absorb.

But a new breed of container ship is now predicted. There is talk of tonnages up to 75,000 d.w.t. in place of the 25,000 d.w.t. of today. *Each mammoth container ship would be capable of carrying as much cargo in a year as an entire fleet of conventional general-cargo carriers.*

Leaving out the difficulties of producing and assembling 75,000 tons of cargo in containers several times a year, and assuming, and indeed it is a major assumption, that it has been successfully shipped, what kind of reception will it get when the ship breaks bulk? Imagine that 25,000 tons consists of whisky—a main currency earner. Hitherto receivers have taken about 1000 tons from each conventional cargo liner. They have storage space and they have their distributive arrangements for coping with this tonnage. What can they be expected to do with arrivals of the order of 25,000 tons if they have built a business based on the weekly arrival of 1000 tons? The wholesaler cannot absorb more than the total of off-licenses that he supplies can take. Space in the shop in the High Street, wherever this may be, is limited to a turnover that has been dictated by the customers. To put the problem crudely, are people who buy, perhaps three bottles a month, going to buy seventy-five bottles because the wholesaler cannot hold the stock? The general reaction would very rightly be "Why tell me?" Stocks of whisky, tobacco, and the like fine cargo cannot be left out in the open where it would be an attraction to evil-minded persons.

When goods are taken out of bond, duty is paid by the importer. Is he going to be able to find the duty on 25,000 tons instead of 1000? It is very unlikely that he will be willing or able, or that it would suit his business to do so. If he cannot pay the duty the goods have got to remain in bonded storage at a high rent. The argument might be put forward: Why not leave several thousand tons of tea or tobacco that the market doesn't want in the containers it came over in? Are containers built to stand up to variations of temperature and humidity for long periods? Not all countries enjoy the temperate conditions that rule in the United Kingdom. In any case, it would not make sense to use transit equipment for storage—about as sensible as using barges for warehousing cargo; all this apart from the tying up of capital.

Many cargoes consist of seasonal crops; in certain areas nature has been persuaded to produce two crops of sugar and rice annually. There is already too much sugar in the world today. The customers for rice consist largely of those poor countries who cannot afford to buy more. In the case of the softwood industry packaging has revolutionized port handling. But this will add marginally, if at all, to the consumption of timber which is largely determined by the building situation. The demand here is governed by the mortgage market which takes no cognisance of how timber is handled in the ports. The cutting, sorting, and preparing for shipment is a complex matter, and the yards that supply the Baltic, Russian, and Canadian exports have been geared to the rather tedious pace set in the past by the handling of softwood loose. On this process the packaging of timber has already made its mark; a level will ultimately be found where fewer ships will be needed in the trade because of the quicker turnround.

If the fact be accepted that the overall tonnage dealt with through ports is not going to be increased, despite the fact that handling in containers is so much faster, then instead of the gradual and continuous process to which we have all become used, we shall have to become accustomed to its absorption by fits and starts. This will produce for the port, not work for 7 days a week, but intermittently, a few hours at a time and this for a very few men. If 75,000-ton container ships were ever to become the pattern of the port, then everyone could go home and wait for the arrival of the same mammoth ship on her next voyage.[1]

How is the port to remain viable if the demands on the facilities it was built to provide are cut back so drastically? Will there be any demand in a few years time for container berths in the enclosed docks? The prototype berths in London and Southampton would be liable to replacement by jetty berths with plenty of background space.

A few years ago a prominent shipowner diagnosed the difficulties of shipping companies as having to buy "the smallest and the slowest ship that will do the job". This is literally true, and it applies to the 75,000-d.w.t. ship as well as to the small coaster. The final problem is presented by the fact that such a ship could by itself carry the tonnage that is now transported by the normal fleet of conventional cargo ships owned and run by a shipping line. It will do this in the four or five voyages that the speedier turnround will permit. Surely the vital process of loading the ship would depend on the importers co-operating to make such a programme possible. Assuming all the practical difficulties have been overcome, the fact remains that the importer will not want the present pattern altered. He is the one with the say-so, and he controls the selection of the ship that will do the job.

It would be a tragedy if these new ships, taking £20 million each to build, had to wait for cargo or travel half-empty because the importer doesn't want the cargo. And how do you make him?

Is the tail in danger of trying to wag the dog?

[1] The fate of the large shore staffs of shipping companies and port authorities that now minister to the wants of the general cargo-ship cannot be lightly dismissed.

Additional Notes

Chapter 10, page 151, par. 1. Roll-on container shipments. The *Atlantic Causeway* with a sister ship to come, belonging to Atlantic Container Line are large roll-on vessels for the North Atlantic service.

Page 158, par. 3. Container flats. These are now being built to a width that will hold two standard Australian pallets.

Page 159, par. 1. In July 1970 this problem had not been finally settled for those depots within 5 miles of the River Thames—container depots.

Page 163, par. 2. Container bridge. The principle of the container bridge has been rejected by the majority of shippers; it is being successfully used in Australia.

CHAPTER 11

MANAGEMENT, STAFF, AND ADMINISTRATION

Introduction

In this survey of some of the conditions that should be present in the efficient port, emphasis is properly placed on the practical or operational side. That does not mean that the managerial and the administrative side can be ignored. The two decades since the Second World War have shown that there is a place in the port for the planner as well as the master stevedore, the thinker of policy as well as the picker-up and putter-down again of cargo units. No port can flourish unless its management has a lively appreciation of the importance of the day-to-day work; no port can continue to function by concentrating all its efforts on the detail of ship and warehouse work. The acceptance of the principle that too much practical experience can be as grave a handicap as too little, was a major step forward in port development.

Function of the Early Ports

To a dock proprietor of half a century ago the fact that his port was not and could never be, an island unto itself, was not allowed to intrude into his main purpose of paying dividends to his shareholders and having enough money over to keep the dock estate in reputable shape, enough to hold his present, and to attract some new, business. It was apparent to few of the pre-1914 dock companies that this was a self-defeating principle. While they were giving, figuratively speaking, their buildings a fresh coat of paint, the river which carried the shipping on which they relied was gradually silting up. Other ports, both in their own and in competitive countries, were attracting new industries and new ideas.

And so the need for a port authority was recognized—a body that would make itself responsible primarily for the port as a port and not as a trading concern. As the years passed, those functions that were not directly remunerative increased. Starting with the most urgent (in many cases)

169

dredging, this led inevitably to river conservation, riparian supervision, and the taking over of powers to regulate and to control river traffic. Coming down to the present day this has led to the installation of radar on a large scale over estuarial waters. Port authorities have waged a war, in which there would seem to be no discharge, against pollution by industrial and municipal effluents.

Government Intervention

Perhaps it was the wholesale scale on which governments had in 1939–45 to plunge into port matters, that finally broke through the iron curtain by which ports had hitherto been surrounded. In a poem written with the background of a similar menace in the First World War, Kipling had commented on the strange spectacle of liners, built for the Far East, carrying troops across the Atlantic, or North American freighters passing through the Suez Canal. Much more so did this become the pattern in the Second World War. Ship diversion was practised to an extent that port operators, used to a set pattern that had identified ports and separate docks with particular ocean spheres, could never have conceived. It was a case of making the available port, or anchorage, fit the available vessel whatever company's flag she might be flying. Many theatres of war outside Europe did not lie alongside areas where first-class ports were waiting to function. If they did, their facilities were the immediate target of enemy aircraft. And so there grew up the acceptance of a new principle—that of overside discharge at a roadstead. True, this had been the working order in some areas off the West African ports or in natural harbours like Hong Kong. Buoy berths were widely used in certain Far Eastern ports, but the discharge of complete expeditionary forces against a peremptory time schedule was a different matter from loading coconuts or logs in the stream. It all helped to breach the wall of convention that had, until then, protected ports from encroachment by new ideas.

Post-war Intervention

Governments having had, willy-nilly, to take ports and their operation and administration under their wing in wartime, would have been very remiss if they had not come to understand the function of a port in the national economy. There were so many jobs that the Government, and they alone, could do. In the United Kingdom a start had been made by grasping the hoary nettle of casual labour. Imperfect both in conception and manipulation, the National Dock Labour Board did mark the biggest step forward in the history of port labour. Unlike many of the wartime schemes it was retained and upon this basis the structure of decasualization was built 20 years later.

What is the total of port facilities in a maritime country? What relation has their distribution to national as opposed to local needs? Are there too many ports and do some still linger on to serve industries, the residue of which could be catered for elsewhere? How often do we find two major ports competing for a traffic that could be economically handled by either? Is there justification for London to have been set up as a passenger port when Southampton, a short train or car journey away, has many obvious advantages? These are but examples of the problems that in a national economy do demand consideration and are outside port prestige and the desire to increase tonnage figures. In short, the days when every port could function, either by expanding or contracting, to suit a policy entirely that of its directors, be they private or municipal, and with the minimum regard to the overall needs of the country, have now gone. Some people think that by nationalization the complete national control of ports will be obtained; this will be discussed later.

That there is room for improvement no one will deny, least of all port proprietors themselves. In the way that it can be brought about, there are as many cures as physicians. There is not even agreement on the diagnosis of the illness. What is the function of a port likely to be in a future domin- ated by containers and the bulk cargo? One of the opposing sides maintains, and can point already to having had some success, that containers can, with some adjustment, be regarded as general cargo as far as their functional handling is concerned. The container and the unit load, they claim, are subservient to the port which, come what may, must retain much of its conventional pattern and must continue to perform many of its traditional functions. The port must remain greater than the cargo it handles.

The other side claim to have taken a longer view of the relation that will emerge eventually between the port and its cargo. To them the container will predominate; general cargo will be so reduced as to have a progressively minor voice in determining the shape and the function of a port. They refuse to have their thinking dominated by the nineteenth-century image of the enclosed, constant-level port, into which container ships will enter, merely because their predecessors for 100 years have done so. They go as far as asserting that a container ship could load at a jetty provided there is an assembly ground sufficiently large in its rear. They consider that the container ship should dominate the port to the extent of ignoring the facilities that the port has always been proud to provide and for which they claim the container ship will have a decreasing need. They point to the labour troubles that have arisen over the staffing of outside container depots as being due entirely to the slavish joining together in thought of ship and cargo. Because exports have, in the docks, always been handled by dockers, and because containers are export cargo, is no reason why the time has not now come for this join-up to be broken down. In this they are undoubtedly right. Since 1945 we have seen so many tribal customs stripped of their warm and conventional clothing and exposed to the hostile blasts of revolutionary ideas. To demote the port from its traditional position of the kingpin in the transportation process to one where the function of transferring goods from sea-borne to land-carriage transport can equally well be done outside its docks, is not likely to commend itself to port authorities generally. There is substance in it, however; the note of economy will insist on being heard.

Types of Port Management

Like so much else concerned with ports, the difficulty when considering management problems, again obtrudes—there is no standard port management from which one can work or to which one can level up. Not only have the demands made on port authorities continually changed in the last century, but they are still a long way from being stabilized. What duties should be undertaken by the port management and which by the port users? There is no agreement on the functions of port authorities even on that most basic of all—who should do the daily work of the master stevedore and the public warehousekeeper? The position is so complex that a logical account of the practices of each major world port would make a jumble of unreadable detail.

This is hardly surprising when a glance is given at the way in which ports have developed. The design of the management structure is largely determined by the port's geographical situation, the industrial and social background, and, not least, the type of goods that are handled. Consider the never-ending problems facing the management in London or Liverpool because they are estuarial ports which have to maintain constant level enclosed docks. Compare their headaches with those of Genoa or Naples where tidal movement can be disregarded and dredging is not a daily chore that can be neglected only at the risk of the approaches to the port silting up. The problems of a port which is ideally situated as a transit centre call for an approach different from the transport centre whose revenue is gained largely from the warehousing and the working of specialized cargoes.

Managements in the ports of West Germany illustrate the extent to which the principle of decentralization of power can operate. Private enterprise shares in the daily work of both Hamburg and Bremen, each of which have their own Free Port. Local authorities in other ports take an active part. In the Low Countries, port activities occupy an important part in the national economy. The general pattern is for local authority to take responsibility for management, with the State taking an active hand in many of the major aspects of port running, including access to the sea and pilotage. At the same time, a port such as Rotterdam has set a world pattern in port development whilst it has succeeded in retaining private enterprise as the dominant factor in running the port.

In the United Kingdom there are four main forms that management has taken. Most important is the Statutory Trust port found in London and Liverpool. A form of management has here been successful for many decades; it is composed of council representatives and the like, plus a majority that represents the users of the port. Where ports are situated on estuaries, the duties include conservancy and the control of shipping moving within the port's limits. Despite the seemingly conflicting interests to be found among the users of the port and the port authority of which they form a part, such as the allocation of master stevedores' duties, there has been no demand to replace this type of management. The daily work is done by a general manager; special committees cover every phase of the work, and there is a chairman and vice-chairman elected by the board, of which they need not be members. Some ports have, since 1948, been nationalized and are run by the British Transport Commission. Of the municipally owned ports, the most important is Bristol. Manchester is run by the Manchester Ship Canal Company.

Conditions in French ports are different. After the French Revolution they became State property coming either under the Ministry of Marine (these having some strategic importance) or the Minister of the Interior. When the Ministry of Works was created, they passed under its control. Since then there have been two forms of management—State ports and self-governing ports. The port director has the responsibility for administration and port running, and he exercises his powers under the minister. In the larger ports he has the services of an advisory committee composed of representatives from local councils, the chambers of commerce, and the users of the port.

Italian ports are, with the exception of Genoa, State owned and are managed by the Ministry of Marine, maintenance and construction works being controlled by the Ministry of Public Works. Genoa is run by an administration council composed of government officials and representatives, from among others, the town councils of Genoa, Milan, and Turin and the chambers of commerce.

In Belgium there is much diversity in the running of their ports. Antwerp, Ghent, and Ostend are municipally owned. The major port, Antwerp, is governed by a council, the daily working being entrusted to a committee of burgomaster and councillors. There is a director-general who is responsible for co-ordinating the various services. Although private enterprise does not take part in the administration of the port, it is responsible for the master stevedoring and this includes the warehousing and dispatch of cargoes, work which would normally be done by the port authority. Zeebrugge belongs to a private firm in which the Belgian Government are interested.

What Ports have in Common

Although there is so much difference in the management basis of the ports of western Europe there is an overriding acceptance today that a port is more than the quays, the berths and the buildings of which it is composed. It is an economic entity. The Second World War demonstrated the strategic importance of ports. They can, if efficiently directed, form the basis of an affluent Society. In an island economy they can be the bottlenecks which negative the higher production achieved inland. Apart from air transport, every package imported or exported has to pass across the quays of an island State. The low priority given to the rebuilding of the national ports of Great Britain, immediately following the extensive damage of the Second World War, was a profound mistake; it illustrated the failure of a government that pressed for exports but had not the knowledge of how the export trade depends always on ports.

With all the in-built diversity that exists between ports, as this brief survey shows, there are certain features and functions that port managements have in common. One of these—the ease with which ships and their cargoes can be diverted from the original destination to a port where labour is willing and ready to load or to discharge the cargo—has recently been demonstrated in the case of strike-prone ports of Great Britain.

Some Duties of Management

Nothing is more striking to the serious student of port development than to note the duties which have, in the last century of working, gradually been accepted by port management as properly coming within their scope. Industrial developments have directly produced new problems, some of which require instant decisions. The serious threat of oil pollution from tankers was mercifully spared the grandparents of present administrators— fortunately, for the only equipment available to them was the frying-pan tied on a broom-handle, and with this they inadequately coped with local slicks of oil escaping from the early oil-burning ships. The regulation of vessels arriving or sailing from a major port has, with the introduction of radar, and the vast improvement in its uses during the last few years, become an important part of the conservancy of the port. Without this the movement of ships, with bulk carriers having apparently no limit to their size, within the narrow and congested estuarial waters would have been done only at great hazard. This movement has been made possible by continuous dredging, done at increasing cost per ton of the spoil removed. All the time there is the problem facing port managements of how far dredging is practicable and for how long the larger vessels will be able to pass through—or may even wish to pass through—the restricted entrances to their docks. The alternative berths for bulk, or container ships must be considered carefully in anticipation of the demand; problems of possible sites, local labour, and in the case of container ships the linkage with container stuffing storage depots, are a few of the problems that are crying out to be solved (Fig. 29).

Reference has already been made to the responsibility of the port authority to provide up-to-date amenities not only for its own workers but other users of the docks. There is a demand, most difficult to determine and to anticipate, from carmen, lightermen, and railway workers. Always there is the probable need during overtime hours of expensive canteen facilities. No private contractor would undertake an enterprise that was expected to serve one or two gangs on a Sunday morning, and without which refreshment the gangs would refuse to work. The standard demanded of washing accommodation, too, is very high; it has been rare

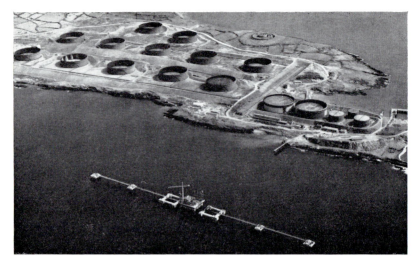

FIG. 29. Bantry Bay, Republic of Ireland, bulk-oil terminal.
(By courtesy of the Ministry of Transport and Power, Republic of Ireland.)

to find a port where the workers have expressed full satisfaction for the amenities provided, most of which they enjoy—and at times abuse—free of charge to themselves.

A weakness in port management that has persisted until the present day is in the system of communications that have kept the upper and the lower tiers of port workers in contact with each other. Until the happenings in United Kingdom ports, following decasualization, pointed to the urgent need to bring all grades into the picture, communication was at a minimum. At the beginning of the century the idea that the executive grades, below the few top rankers, should be allowed to know the management's plans for the future, or even to sense the thinking that would determine these, would certainly not have been entertained. Knowledge of this kind was the privilege of the few. "It is not a good thing for the staff to know too much", dismissed the question for another decade. Management, when the future of some section of the staff was at stake and it was pressed, with deference and politeness, to disclose some of its plans, took refuge in phrases such as "the time is not opportune" or "our plans would be prejudiced by premature disclosure". Several major ports have not discarded completely these moth-eaten garments that protected management from what was regarded as the curiosity of underlings. Today's changes, urged on port authorities by the container and the bulk load, the closing down of whole dock systems, the making redundant of whole classes of the staff, are so sweeping that it is good common sense to tell the staff what is going to happen and to deal with their reasonable doubts.[1] Seen against the domestic background of the workers, the threat to his job is a far more real thing than the mark on the planners' paper. Nothing travels round a port quicker than rumour, and the grapevine has a prolific and often malevolent growth. It is management's job to put over the idea that the worst never happens before "for every bad there is a worse" idea takes hold.

Communications can best be improved not by one man but by dock managers and heads of departments. They should have regular meetings with their staff and labour, showing an appreciation of the doubts and difficulties that the present unsettled times in dockland are producing. For labour to realize that their opinions are valuable, for the staff to be told that the routine work they do matters a great deal, all this is re-assuring in an industry where few are at present without their doubts as to their personal future.[2]

The limited experience already gained at berths where the piecework scramble and the daywork dawdle have been replaced by the team that "belongs" to the berth, illustrates forcibly how men who have been made part of the team react to this new approach. Brought up to expect the big stick, they saw, after 1945, this traditional method replaced by the big shilling. Neither threats nor appeasement have been successful as a basis for dock labour relations. All they have produced is "us or them", with the team spirit further away than before. The astounding turnround times at berths that are operated by an appeal to technical skill and craftmanship encourage both sides to extend what is really an exercise in communications.

Management is today required to take a much wider view of its re-sponsibilities than did its predecessors. Every port is concerned with opera-tional developments, not only those taking place in its sister ports but also those in other countries. Nearly all ports are today competitive. There is

[1] A major managerial problem that is now emerging is the loss of morale due to staff dissatisfaction with the high wages that labour is now getting compared with their own salaries; this combined with the opportunities of promotion which get less with every dock closure.
[2] A lead has been given in making communications within the port a personal matter between management, staff, and labour by the Port of London Authority.

no final pattern of what each port does or will do should its rivals fall down on some branch of their activities. The increasing traffic that has been won by small ports from the major ports, their very existence hardly noticed a decade ago, will be commented on later. Labour agreements are normally made on national bases; some are made for a specific purpose such as the West Coast Agreement in the United States, and subsequent labour charters, all of which affect, and may require careful study by, ports in other countries.

Problems Within the Port

The fundamental fact that a port exists to make a profit cannot be ignored. A glance at the plan of a 100-year-old dock will show that 95 per cent of the buildings and installations that figure therein were there to produce revenue. Many of those that have now gained a place within the dock estate are non-productive. They are necessary within the changed pattern of dock working but they produce no revenue. It is as well that this fact should predominate and should control experiments that, however attractive they may seem, may cost more than the revenue they bring in.

Among the duties that port authorities have undertaken have been surveys on traffic flows. Perhaps more pertinent is the continual search for improvement in the operational methods by which the daily movement of cargoes—the essential picking up and putting down again—is performed. Nothing has determined these methods more than custom and practice. Agreements made for certain cargoes to be handled in certain ways are up to date when they are made. In half a century they can have become completely obsolete without the port authority noticing this. A few pertinent "why's" will reveal that the conditions against which the agreement was first made have now disappeared.

The documentation that originally intended to speed up the movement of cargo had, by the 1950s, succeeded almost in strangling it. To leave the port of New York, it was reported, some 1000 pieces of paper for one ship and her cargo had to be prepared, under complex rules that were known only to a few specialist firms. Fowarding agents make a living by mastering the idiotic requirements of their national Customs, often incomprehensible to the firms that ship the cargo. Air freight, sensibly, would have none of this. To the consternation of the babu mind that motivates officialdom, cargoes were moved by air—safely and ten times more speedily without the documents that smothered the movement of a single package by sea across the English Channel. The documentary system of every maritime country had been born of ignorance and suspicion. It was erected over the centuries to protect the shipper from the mentality of the smuggler and the pirate. Every party that had a hand in the movement of cargo was suspect and was thought, sometimes correctly, to have designs on the goods. Claims for losses, shortages, and damages were an accepted nightmare. The staff maintained by port authorities and shipping companies to contest these, cost more than it would have done to pay them, as was quickly found by ports which, after 1945, had the courage to abolish, or to modify, the tallying of cargo. Staff engaged in preventing losses, the bulk of which have proved to be imaginary, do not earn revenue. Their justification would be if they saved more than they cost. At the conservative figure of 2s. (10p) a ton for tallying today it is worth the attention of port management, whether this is, in fact, so.

To deal with cargo passing over the quays of two ports in Great Britain, $1\frac{1}{4}$ million documents a year, it is stated, are required. As many as sixty entries on various forms and records were needed for some individual consignments. To Sweden the world owes the initiative in cutting down the number of documents and the time and money wasted on their preparation. The steps taken by Swedish exporters in 1955 were copied by their neighbours in Denmark. In 1961 the United Nations Economic Committee for Europe invited each country to tackle the problem, and this resulted in the United Kingdom in the publication in 1965 of *Simpler Export Documents*. The basic idea behind these improvements was the preparation of a set of documents all printed on the same size paper, ranging from the bill of lading through to Lloyd's insurance certificate, on which information common to all is reproduced in the same relative position. This had the immediate effect of standardizing the form and size of the bill of lading and the export note.

Despite the lip service paid to standardization of shipping documents, it is a fact that the man who introduces a new form meets with less opposition than he who attempts to abolish an existing one. A large proportion of clerical staff—and this includes high officials—earn a living by juggling with the information provided on forms. It is expecting too much, however, that officials so occupied should show enthusiasm for abolishing the means that produce their daily bread. This, however, does not apply to port managements. They have noted the steady progress that has slowly and painstakingly been made, and they have appreciated the savings that have overlapped on to their own working. Some have adopted the standard A4 paper for their own relevant documents. There is room for a close scrutiny, a justification for every form that is in daily use within their undertaking. Staff should be forbidden to invent a new form without authority from the top.

How will the container affect the number of forms still in use? It is naturally hoped that the marked increase in the size of the unit load will lead to a decrease in their number. If the traffic should eventually settle down into a pattern where a single transport agency carries a container from door to door, there will be scope. It must be borne in mind that the inland depot will take the place, from the all-important point of liability, of what is colloquially called "the ship's rail". The exporter will lose control of his goods, not at the export shed door but at a depot some miles inland. Similarly, the importer will not accept liability, as hitherto, at the tail board of his collecting lorry, but at this same depot. It is here that the activities of the national Customs will commence. Shipping and forwarding agents, struggling to keep pace with the ever-growing demands for information about consignments they handled, were grateful for the week or so that the average export vessels took to load. It gave them the time for the documents "to do the rounds" and to be forwarded in time to catch up with the goods. With container ships loading and discharging in a matter of hours they have been deprived of this period of grace. A joint approach by shipping companies and officials of the Customs service has been made in the face of so active a threat. It meant that all the benefits of containerization achieved at so great a cost could be nullified by the absence of a piece of paper.

Perhaps the most direct line on which savings can be made by simplifying internal work, is an overhaul of the port's system of dues on ships and charges on goods. The size and complexity of these will be determined by the overall functions exercised by the management. If it is responsible for the daily work, for the discharge of cargoes, the assembly and tendering to the shipping company of all exports that pass across the quays, and for the warehousing and the complying with trade requirements of specialized imports, then its pile of rate schedules will, over the years, have mounted up. If it fulfils only the function of a landlord, it will be that much less.

The first object of a charges system—a convenient term to include the varied forms into which the tariff structure has proliferated through many generations—is to make possible the collection of revenue. This should be sufficient in amount to pay labour and staff directly responsible for producing revenue; also it must cover the payment of non-revenue earning staff. On top of these direct demands there is a host of claims on revenue that may extend from the purchase of rat poison to the payment of staff pensions. Basically, the charges for services on goods should be related to the cost of paying productive staff and labour. Before 1939 it was appreciated by port officers responsible for departmental work that their costs should never be more than 50 per cent of the revenue their department earnt; every 10s. (50p) they spent should bring in £1 to the port authority. Recently a major port authority has admitted that it now costs them 14s. 10d. (74p) to earn £1.

With the rapidly changing face of cargo presentation and handling, a system of charges that satisfied the static traffic of the inter-war years is no longer of use. Tremendous improvements in the handling of unit loads and bulk cargoes have enabled reduced charges to be quoted, thus attracting more traffic to the port that is efficient enough to employ them. By adhering to the principle that charges must be related directly to costs and that these may be expected to be in inverse relation to the size of the cargo unit—it costs the same for a crane to lift a package of one hundred-weight as one ton—they have succeeded in reducing their export schedule, containing 2000 rates, to a mere dozen, and a schedule of port rates from 4300 to less than 240.

Granted that charges should be based on costs, there is some room for so framing a tariff that encouragement is actively given to the shipper and the importer to review the method of presentation and the packaging of his cargoes. Port authorities who have bought expensive handling equipment can never slacken in their attempts to gain traffic suitable for the machines they now own. It has long been accepted that a direct saving on terminal costs will appeal more to the user of the port than government exhortations. They will listen to the port authority speaking to them through the columns of their rate book.

Organization and Method

As a precursor of today's elaborate system of surveys, consultancies, and computers, the O & M branch of a port authority can be credited with having done good work. Basically it set out to cover ground that had been regarded as the prerogative of the general manager, but which he had neither the time nor the detailed knowledge to cover. The early attempts, some of which dated from the years immediately after the First World War, under the general and rather vague name of "research", were often handicapped by the personality of the officers seconded to the job; also by a general and understandable opposition of departmental heads who saw research proposals as a direct encroachment on their powers. "Good ideas" appealed only to the inventor, who consistently failed to enlist the enthusiasm of those on whom he depended to carry them out. The general manager foresaw friction among the departments if he attempted to carry out research ideas. He had some reason to doubt the claims that were made for the savings that would result. No head of a port authority will welcome progress if this is another name for inter-departmental troubles which can very easily arise between senior officers. There was often the suspicion that research, in order to secure a few good marks, had put forward proposals without sufficient inquiry or had failed to master the complexities that underlie all major dock jobs.

Therefore the officer in charge of O & M must have the right personality. He must be identified with the port authority and not with any part of it. He must be acceptable to the engineering staff; his work must be done in a leisurely way with no rushing to conclusions.

Whilst O & M are not concerned with national labour agreements or terms of employment, they will find ample scope for asking "Why?" in the documentary, administrative, or operative work of a port authority. The customs of the port and traditional methods of doing certain jobs will keep a conscientious O & M department profitably occupied. The actual day-by-day employment of staff, the continuous asking "Why do you do that?" or "Why is it done that way?" can yield surprising results.

A New Conception of a Port Authority

Under the heading of "Training and developing human skills as a condition for technical innovation and organizational change",[1] an examination has been made of training by management—not of technical skills at workers' and staff level—but rather as a development of technical, social, and conceptual skills at all levels. It is claimed that these problems are now topical in Dutch ports, and although there must be many ports

[1] Dr. A. H. Bos, Management Development Consultant, Holland, in a paper read to the International Cargo Handling Co-ordination Association's Technical Conference, Gothenburg, June 1969.

that have not yet reached a level where serious consideration can yet be given them, the time when this will be so is rapidly approaching.

The Present demands dynamism and creativity. While the transport world has been involved later than other industries, this makes it possible to profit from the experience of others. Management by intuition must give way to the three tasks of creating markets, managing the means of production, and developing human capacities, the whole related to the port and its facilities. Firstly, management must decide—in the light of the urgent need to make a profit—the objectives of the enterprise, and these must be pursued with a singleness of purpose. Secondly, in doing just this, the improvisation that has hitherto served must give way to scientific management as expressed in the various accepted aspects of planning. The uncertain and largely unpredictable nature of dockwork have made difficult such an approach hitherto. More of the management's attention must be given to internal organization questions, and in this O & M will doubtless have a part to play.

The development of human capacities, a subject that in port circles can hardly be claimed as being topical, has already been touched upon under the heading of communications. This, however, goes no further than keeping staff and labour advised of present change and future planning. It does little to consider the worker as other than being concerned with his pay packet and, probably, the security of his job.

Both policies of the big stick and the big shilling are built on the assumption that the worker has no desire to take a part in the enterprise that fills his pay packet. It has been possible, through piecework and bonus systems, to get a satisfactory performance, but this satisfaction—on both sides—has never been permanent. Whilst positive co-operation is essential, unwillingness to work, or work frustration in its many forms, has been only too apparent. Port work as expressed in the container berth or the berth serving an integrated industry, calls for a positive co-operation from all workers. To bring out this willingness, to replace the mutual suspicion and the catch-as-catch-can attitude, inseparable from the present system, is not impossible. The suggestion made in some cases by labour, of the team basis on a selected berth, is a healthy sign that higher wages are linked with a desire for co-responsibility of the workers. The team idea sprang from a realization by a few forward-looking dockers that they were getting nowhere by making a series of demands, each more exorbitant than the last. Trade was being lost to competitive ports—it could be seen to be lost. The only way to recover some of this, and to gain new trade, was by letting the world of shipping see that the men on the team berth were there to co-operate. The idea that inspired the team was exactly what the management had longed for but never dared to expect—that the docker should come to the dock to work irrespective of the daily difficulties and the "book".

Asked recently what was the secret of his contentment, despite long hours of work and incessant travel, the head of an international combine expressed it as "belonging". His work was accepted and appreciated by his co-equals; he belonged to a most exclusive set, entry to which could be gained by merit only. Will it be possible to induce this esoteric feeling among port workers or is this beyond the horizon of port management? There is increasing recognition that the "economic man" of the nineteenth century is an out-of-date phenomenon. The threat of unemployment which inspired the urge to better oneself is no longer present. Can it be replaced, gradually no doubt, and over the course of a decade or two, by the worker who "belongs" to his industry and takes the same pride in doing so as does his general manager in the more rare atmosphere that he breathes.

Port operators who recollect the tough inter-war years, will not take kindly to the use of the word "spiritual" as applying to the worker's attitude to his job. It has been defined as the challenge that all men seek—and often fail to find—in their job. This has been found to be particularly present in young workers. If it can be encouraged and exploited, management will gain workers who have learnt to stand on their own feet, to take decisions on their own, and to accept responsibility as new challenges come along. They will have gained for themselves and for the port for which they work that invisible but priceless asset, the "know-how", a quality that every port has to a differing extent. When it has sunk below a certain level the worker, it has been found, becomes averse to taking responsibility, withdraws into the daydreams of the routine worker, or alternatively employs his energy by aggressive opposition to management. This deadly process follows on his realization that his employer has no interest in him as a fellow worker, does not look out for or expect his co-operation, nor provides any opportunity by way of challenges in the work on which he can exercise his innate skill. It is a mistake, and the experience of every service officer confirms this, to work on the principle that the capacity to co-operate, to take decisions, and to accept respon- sibility is not present. It is far easier to assume that the worker wants (and this may find expression in the most simple forms) to develop his talents through his work. This is present through the need of most workers to gain the respect of their mates through the quality of their daily work. The next and more satisfying stage is to have gained the respect of the employer through the co-operation which has been built up by attending to the spiritual side of the contract.

Additional Notes

Chapter 11, page 178, par. 4. Simplified rating. The PLA has now replaced fourty-four Import Schedules on Imported Goods with one publication of 44 pages.

Page 178, par. 4. SITPRO. The International Chamber of Commerce formed, in 1969, the Joint Advisory Committee on Simplification and Standardization of External Trade Documents, now functioning as SITPRO.

Page 180, par. 2. Standardized shipping note. The PLA have produced a simple standard shipping note; failure by shippers and others to use this adds to the terminal charges imposed.

CHAPTER 12

THE PORT OF THE FUTURE

Introduction

Since 1945 the accepted pattern of our ports has been completely upset. Experts admit that the future shape of the industry is by no means clear. Already in New York there are serious problems due to the drying up of the traditional break-bulk handling centres and the turning over to the unit load, the container, and bulk traffic. This disturbing movement has spread to ports in Great Britain and Europe. Neither employers nor labour can stand in the way of this trend. From being an industry whose problems could be solved by applying more and better labour, it is becoming increasingly recognized that bigger and better mechanical equipment to handle the larger units that now present themselves for shipment, with fewer demands on port labour, will give the answer in the future.

There is a school of thought that believes that by the year 2000 the freight-carrying ship with which, in its various forms, generations have been familiar, will be a picturesque survival. Cargo will be carried in atomic-powered submersible ships independent of weather and surface conditions and discharged by helicopters or barges detached from the deck of a super surface liner at a huge floating terminal. Such advanced ideas smack too much of science fiction to be developed here. An examination of the way that ports can, in the year 1969, be seen to be developing is a more practical way of tackling the subject. It is certain that building bigger and better berths of the conventional pattern is now outside practical politics. Construction of special berths is proceeding apace; there is no certainty that they will be contained within the enclosed dock. It has long been accepted that no two ports run in identical lines; it is just possible that in the future United Kingdom and European ports, for instance, will become increasingly dependent on each other. The refusal in 1969 of London dockers to handle containers for Australia and their shipment to north European ports for shipment there, is an instance of this new dependence.

In the past the importance of ports has been shown by the concentration of a great deal of activity in a relatively small area. Other links in the transportation chain were apt to be overshadowed. With modern developments, including the far less spectacular internal movement of containers, the place that the port will occupy in the whole process of transportation will be less easy to define where the efficiency of all is in question. The quicker turnround of shipping will continue to be important, but once a container service becomes established, port processes—the subject of so much heated discussion during the last two decades—will become very much routine and not capable of further improvement.[1] There will certainly be concentration on cargo that cannot be carried in containers as well as on those ports that are not suitable for container handling. Palletization and forklift trucks will be used to solve many of these problems: excellent results have already been obtained from fully automatic computerized warehouses, particularly for chests of tea which can be piled fifteen high, in prepared stowage racks. The need for publicizing the facilities that the port can provide, the opportunities for development that it can produce, and the details of the daily cargo receiving position for each vessel loading, have been recognized. The function of the inland port has not yet been defined, but it is significant that inland cargo terminals where only the ship is missing, have been discussed both in northern Italy and in Switzerland. Nearness of the port to the industrial area is always a contributory reason for its development: the gigantic new harbour being built in the Gulf of Fos, on the south coast of France, will lead to the establishment of several new industrial zones within the area. The Victorian convention that something would be done about new berths only after the trade had come knocking on the port's doors has given way to the anticipation of demand after close research has been made into possible cargo patterns of the future. It has been found that by creating the facilities in advance of the demand, a demand for these has been created.

---

[1] A new Australian container service will operate from the summer of 1970 that will represent the present entire national liner interest in the trade of Britain, France, Germany and the Netherlands. Fourteen big container ships will become a single fleet with integrated operations, pooled revenues, and a single sales and marketing organization in each European country. These will be sufficient to carry the entire trade (plus a few Scandinavian and break-bulk vessels) with regular sailings and common documentation. (*The Times*, 27 October 1969.)

Containers—Their Effect on Ports

This aspect of port development so overshadows all others that we make no apology for returning to it. The future of every major and most small ports depends largely on the position they will eventually be able to establish as main or feeder ports. As a third role they may do very well as a terminal for coastwise or near-continental container shuttle services. The facilities they may be able to offer for the establishment and the working of container depots will be important. It should not be lost sight of that a successful container traffic presupposes ample industry working near the port and providing a volume of goods that will ensure a continuous two-way traffic. As already emphasized, containers are meant to handle existing demands for goods: they do not, nor can they ever, create a demand.

Not only will container ships spend less time in port but, owing to their larger carrying capacity as compared with general-cargo ships, there will be fewer ships in the port of the future. By making use of feeder ports when the present uncertain position is resolved, shipowners will concentrate on as few ports as possible.[1] The round voyage from Sydney to London, which used to take about 120 days, will be accomplished in about 60 days. As the volume of world cargo to be carried increases, it will be handled so much more efficiently that fewer ships will do the job than are now needed for a smaller tonnage. The alternative will be that many of the existing fleet of container ships will be laid up.

Many experts believe that the ironing out of the present difficulties, in an endeavour to equate the supply and demand for container traffic, will take many years; substantially longer than would a couple of years ago have been predicted. Parallel with this process is the study now going on of berth utilization for general-cargo vessels. This has been made necessary by the quicker ship turnround of break-bulk cargo. Whilst containers have stolen the limelight in the last decade, the discharge and loading of the conventional cargo vessel has steadily improved in terms of gang-hour tonnage. Ports are still bedevilled by their ancient enemies—weather, uncertainties of conditions overseas, politics, and finance, but the container ship and the improved turnround of other ships has helped to iron out the alternation of booms and slumps which was the accepted background

[1] See footnote 1, p. 187. It is expected that between three and four ports only in Europe will be used and three only in Australia.

in the past to all port work. Also the total number of labourers required will so decrease that housing developments for workers in the dock vicinity will not continue to be a major problem. A few years ago an attempt to develop the dock system in London on ground bought for that purpose over half a century earlier was objected to by the local authority because housing for the influx of workers following on the opening of a new dock in outer London could not be coped with. With the notion that ports should spread down the estuary if they wish to survive, it is perhaps fortunate that the PLA did not pour capital into a new dock complex, parts of which have since been closed as obsolete, and while the axe is still suspended over its neighbour next down the River Thames.[1]

The physical position of ports is becoming increasingly important. Southampton, as mentioned already, is now, in regard to container trade, enjoying the advantages with which Bristol was presented when at the end of the fifteenth century its windows opened on to the newly discovered continent of North America.[2] Not to be left behind, London has turned its back on the origin of its power and influence, the nearness of its docks to the Metropolis; it is concentrating not only on Tilbury, 26 miles below the early docks built within sight of London Bridge, but it is extensively investigating the area around Foulness, where docks in deep water could form part of a new complex that will include an airport, oil installations, and other industrial users.[3]

In May 1967 the Mersey Docks and Harbour Board announced plans for a £45 million man-made island, some 3800 ft long for mammoth tankers. The island would be 11 miles from the mainland and in the form of a breakwater to be linked by submarine pipelines to the regional oil refineries. With a depth of 95 ft of water the largest tankers yet contemplated could be berthed, and a turnround time of 24 hours is predicted. Not only could the project provide the most important oil terminal with storage and transhipment facilities in Europe, but it is further indication of the development of ports outside the enclosed docks (Fig. 30 shows a man-made island, Robert's Bank, Vancouver).

[1] At the time of writing (December 1969) the closing of the Surrey Commercial Docks in the port of London is under active consideration.
[2] The combined effect of containerization, new motorways, and freight liner trains has smashed the argument that London and Liverpool enjoyed extensive industrial hinterlands. With modern road and rail developments all the main ports are easily reached.
[3] Rotterdam plans a four-fold increase in trade in the next 20 years.

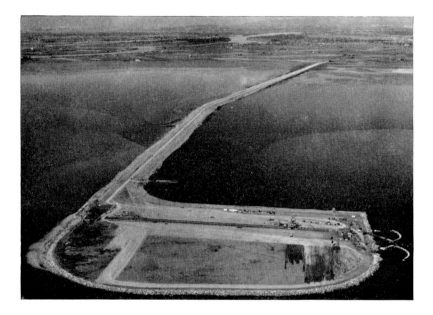

FIG. 30. Man-made island, Robert's Bank, Vancouver, created from dredged material and with a 3-mile long causeway. Ready for the installation of bulk-coal-handling facilities. (By courtesy of the National Harbours Board, Vancouver.)

Redundant Dockers

There seems no alternative to the process, already well under way, of remoulding dock labour from the huge force of semi-skilled labourers into a smaller, mobile,[1] and highly technical body of men with a concentration of port facilities in smaller areas. There may be room for a free port, with its obvious advantages. The example set by Antwerp in developing industries within the perimeter of the dock estate—the integrated port—has been accepted as one important aspect of port development. The competition that now exists among continental ports has been summed up by an official of the Marseilles Port Authority in a minimum of words: "this

[1] The mobile work force, consisting of a body of men, that serves the needs of neighbouring ports where, perhaps, only one container ship arrives weekly, is already in operation in Tasmania. Despite union opposition the idea may be expanded.

is a race, nothing short of that. If we are first we get the business. If we are second we get less business. If we don't do anything we get nothing. Unless we improve and expand we shall be out-of-date."

The important part that hovercraft could play, particularly the large freight-carrying type, in making export traffic more flexible—and this is receiving government interest in respect of their use on short sea routes—calls attention to the basic requirements of a "hoverport" in the development of the port of the future. The place of discharge and loading should be as near as possible to the metropolitan area, it should have good road and rail access and the approach from the beach should be clear of the traditional shipping lanes. Cross traffic in cargo, as between hovercraft and normal shipping, should be minimal. The noise factor calls for consideration also; the slope of the beach is important.

All this terminal business means that the port authority must spend money on research and that this must be of the practical kind, in close liaison with the operating staff. They are the men who control dock operations and on whose shoulders lie the responsibility for turning ideas into successful projects. This should include amenities for labour and for other users of the docks. The excuse that conditions of the work make legislation for providing amenities so much more difficult than the settled conditions of factories, must no longer be made. Within this sphere comes the approach of the port authority to accident prevention. Apart from the humanitarian angle it does not make sense economically to have a proportion of workers permanently prevented from working, by accidents that could, by education and training, be avoided.

The Pattern of the Future

The most logical way of discerning this pattern is to examine the predictable future of the component parts of the present port. How, for instance, will lighterage fare? Before 1939 the trade of the estuarial port, and this applied with some force to the Rhine complex, might consist of as much as 80 per cent of the port's tonnage handled overside. As conditions then were, the remaining 20 per cent was about as much as the shore facilities of the port could handle; the turnround of shipping with an outlet on both sides was far more flexible than in those ports, and they will always exist, where all cargo, in both directions, passes across the quay. It is a fact that the advent of containers has not been matched by equally thrusting methods from the lighterage industry. In many cases it is still handicapped by a system that is only just beginning to show signs of realizing the importance of larger barges.

A radical change in craft design will be required before the lighterage trade can have a part in the container traffic. Barges with a flat deck, accessible to heavy capacity forklift trucks, will be needed where containers can move horizontally on and off. For such craft, pusher tugs would be necessary also. One expert envisages the loading and unloading of containers into hovercraft from a vessel working in the mouth of the estuary. This would imply that the parent ship could remain at sea for years at a time. There are, however, too many practical and human problems to be solved before the modern container ship becomes a twentieth-century *Flying Dutchman*.

The LASH[1] system is the brightest star that the trade at present can contemplate. To take London, for many years a typical lighterage-dominated port, it is sad to see, in the last decade, that the tonnage carried by craft has fallen from 21 million to $5\frac{1}{2}$ million tons and the lighterage force from 5000 to 2000 men. Concurrently, many of the wharves to which barges constantly plied have closed down, as the whole pattern of the industry has altered. In October 1969 there were fourteen LASH ships on order for United States shipping companies.[2] The increasing acceptance of the LASH concept both here and abroad holds out the best prospect for a revival of freighting by barge. As ports tend to expand down river and even to man-built islands some miles off the coast, goods can be carried cheaply and efficiently with a crew of two men taking care of 1000 tons plus of cargo.

How will railways fare? The conventional system of shunting relatively small cargo units, in the form of loaded rail wagons, is ineffective and uneconomic. It will be replaced, and one port has already taken the decision to close its system of more than 100 miles in favour of the establishment within the port area of a railway terminal for freight liner trains. Containers will be lifted off at this point and transferred by road tractor and trailer to the loading berth and vice versa. As the volume of rail traffic has gone steadily down in the last 15 years, the future of rail operations within the port will be limited to the working of specialized transit

---

[1] This is one of five known systems which are described in a paper read at New York in September 1969. For a summary see *ICHCA Journal* for November 1969.

[2] The first of these, the *Acadia Forest* (43,000 d.w.t.), arrived in the Thames for discharge on 4 December 1969.

for a particular traffic such as bulk grain. That the decline in rail traffic is fairly general is shown by the drop in rail-borne exports and imports in the port of New York; in 1964 this had dropped to 42·8 per cent of the 1940 figure. Dock railways are expensive in terms of capital investment, maintenance, and the large areas required for their operation.

Whatever changes take place in the pattern of port traffic they should have very little effect on the roads that feed the port. This contribution is a small additional percentage when the port is in a heavily industrialized and populous area. Even with the increased tonnage that container traffic will bring, and assuming that a container berth will have a throughput ten times that of a general cargo berth, the road users will be large lorries of a uniform pattern instead of the assortment of vehicles of many shapes and sizes. If container berths can work on shifts, then pressure on the roads will be spread over a longer period. The demands that will be made on the roads in the container age will not be in proportion to the increase in the volume of traffic.

Port authorities everywhere will be concerned at the land needed for future developments. First reactions to containers envisaged an average of 20 acres per berth. On the one hand, it was emphasized that this would cope with the tonnage normally handled at three general berths. On the other hand, it is not now accepted that containers need to be placed in single tiers over a wide area. They can be piled on the container park already described. The container berth will then need no more space than does the conventional ship. Acquiring land on a large scale for future development may seem a prudent policy, but capital is tied up for many years.

In 1954 the number of loaded vehicles that used services across the English Channel was 506. In 10 years this had gone up to more than 17,000 and the increase continues. Documentation has certainly been simplified by new methods. According to British Customs, hold-ups in traffic could be greatly reduced if there was a higher standard of accuracy in the preparation of Customs documents.

Port Viability

Perhaps the most difficult of all port developments to predict is staff responsibilities in the near future. The present pattern has been built up over the centuries; the relation in numbers between staff of different grades and the labour that does the work has been accurately worked out.

When it is exceeded it can be seen to have done so and is generally cut back. Now there is everywhere a reduction in the amount of labour required; there is no foreseeable end to this process. The supervision required for the loading and unloading of a 25,000-d.w.t. container ship is minimal compared with the small army of foremen and tally clerks needed before 50,000 tons of general cargo could pass over the quays. Conventional practice has always demanded a quota of higher executive and managerial types. With a complex system of charges on goods and dues on ships, a staff of experts was permanently employed unravelling their own rate books. For the same tonnage carried in containers, no staff of this kind would be needed. As more shipping is operated outside the enclosed dock, the services of a dockmaster and his staff will become a luxury too expensive to continue. Will the dock engineer need his present staff to handle the much simpler demands of a container berth? Will the dock police require the same force to guard a non-vulnerable tonnage in containers?

A start has already been made (October 1969) in recognizing and coping with the problem of redundancy among white-collar workers. The aim of one major port is to reconstruct their present staff by streamlining it gradually to a more highly paid but technically more adept staff; it would be brought down to the lower number needed by severance payments akin to those nationally adopted for labour, a cessation of recruitment, and earlier pensions.

General Points

The port of the future will contain few of the features that have been familiar to so many generations. Quay sheds will almost entirely disappear as the need for sorting individual units to marks and quality goes. Sorting, which deters mechanical handling and acts as a brake on speedy turn-round, will be done before loading as is the sorting to sizes of softwood timber now done on the other side before shipment and prior to packaging. The small-capacity quay cranes that spend so much of their lives idle, should disappear.[1] With container vessels and bulk cargoes they should be an anachronism. The overhead gear that many container ships will carry would be able to work cargo during rain when plastic tents could be easily placed over a working hold.

---

[1] A loss on their crane division by a large engineering production company was reported in October 1969.

It is not to be expected that the size of ships will stand still. 1967 saw the second closing of the Suez Canal in 11 years. Even before this plans for the giant tanker on the Kuwait–Bantry Bay run were well advanced. Compared with ships of a size that could negotiate the Canal, the cost of shipping oil in mammoth ships round the Cape was about one-half. In October 1968 the *Universe Ireland* of 312,000 d.w.t., the first of a fleet of six, made her maiden voyage to Bantry Bay. This was selected because it enjoys, permanently, the advantage of having 100 ft of water at 1200 ft from the shore, is an open port for 24 hours a day all the year round, and has the lowest incidence of fog of any port of the north-west European coast. It will be used regularly also for 250,000-d.w.t. tankers.

The super tanker concept is affecting all the major ports of Great Britain and north-west Europe. Finnart, in Western Argyll in Scotland, could take tankers of 200,000 d.w.t. Thameshaven (206,000 d.w.t.) and the Humber are preparing to take mammoth ships. Plans are being studied for the building of an artificial island to take 500,000 d.w.t. ships in the English Channel. The economic use of the giant tanker is closely tied in with further development of ports everywhere. Although not so spectacular, similar strides have been made for other than oil carriers. British Transport Docks Board are providing facilities at both their Humber and South Wales ports for bulk carriers up to 150,000 d.w.t. for high-grade ores for the British Steel Corporation. The size of loose-timber carriers has always been determined by the known slowness of discharge and the acceptance of the inevitable demurrage. With the coming of packaged timber it has been found possible to build ships of some 17,000 d.w.t., more than twice the size of the largest loose-timber carrier that would be tolerated.

Ship speed has not escaped attention. The gap between the 25-knot container ship and the 400 m.p.h. air freight is too great to be ignored. Water transport has always been the slowest, albeit the most dependable, method of getting goods in large quantities from A to B. In 10 years' time we are promised the 100-knot an hour "container air bubble ship" suitable for the North Atlantic service. Cutting down voyage time so drastically could add to the insoluble problems of the 75,000-d.w.t. container ship already discussed.

Dredging, particularly of special channels and port areas, will be increasingly important as ship sizes increase. Tankers of 500,000 d.w.t. will, it is estimated, have a draught of 100 ft. It is satisfactory to note that there will be sufficient depth both in the Straits of Dover and the North Sea (something that has never before been questioned) for these ships. The fact that a minimum of 100 ft might be required in the approaches to a port will make it essential to be certain that there is no underwater obstruction. Where the coast is rocky, sunken rocks, known to exist at this depth, will obtrude into the picture. So also will the continued suitability of the route that has always sufficed. If a 475,000-d.w.t. tanker, contemplated (October 1969) by the United States Caltex Petroleum Corporation, is built, it will have a draught of close on 100 ft. The question may arise whether a ship with this draught could pass safely through the Straits of Malacca on its way from the Persian Gulf to Japan. This may be typical of the precautions that will certainly have to be taken before the oil-hungry areas of Asia can be satisfied.

One method of avoiding off-shore dangers of this kind is to moor the tanker to a buoy anchored in the sea bottom. Cargo is discharged through floating hose which connects the ship to the buoy and then to a shore-bound pipeline.

The work of the International Standards Organization in respect of container sizes has been mentioned. This is now being followed up by the attempt to get a measure of standardization for the equipment used in cargo handling. Inquiries so far made by the British Standards Institution's Advisory Committee on Materials Handling, in conjunction with the Féderation Européene de la Manutention (FEM) and other relevant bodies, cover the operating work done by twenty-one appliances and articles of equipment from aerial ropeways to forklift trucks. Good progress has already been made, and it is hoped that full co-operation of manufacturer and user with the BSI will be attained. The huge sums that were wasted in industry before the nut could be made to fit the bolt should be avoided in the fast-growing business of cargo handling.

It is now better understood that, before full advantage can be taken of mechanization, a new relation between employers and labour must be forged. This will prove to be the most difficult of all problems. There is agreement that piecework is no longer applicable to modern conditions. Its replacement by one general rate with perhaps six variations for difficult or dirty cargoes has been suggested. This would, and both sides must be aware of it, leave the ground open for the continuous disputes over conditions that have marked the work in the port of Liverpool.

Even labour has admitted the futility of running so huge an industry with equipment that is idle for two-thirds of each of the five working days that now make up the working week. Opposition to a shift system has not yet been overcome despite the fact that every week brings evidence of business leaving ports that cling, not only to the old ways of working but, to the old ways of thinking. "Them and us" has no place in the second half of the twentieth century; it continues to dominate ports in some countries. It has been suggested that many of the present troubles could be avoided if there was one union having the sole duty of looking after dockers' interests, which at present are only too often a section, and not an important one, of a mammoth union. However, not even the most forward-looking docker can see such a desirable move as practical save by the intervention of the government of the day.

As far as there is agreement on removing the present causes by which the industry is torn asunder, it is to be found in worker participation; that is, by trade union officials taking part in management. How this will operate in the day-by-day working is not clear; neither are its advocates deterred by the lack of success that has attended the limited spheres in which it has, so far, been tried. Practical participation by the younger dockers has been summarized as the replacement of piecework by the team and better training facilities.

Air Freight

A cloud, once no bigger than a man's hand, is now making its presence felt. The loss of cargo to air freight will be a major concern of the port of the future. The advantages are so obvious that they need no emphasis; it is enough to record the speed at which it has grown. In 1968 airports in the United Kingdom alone handled imports to the value of £1058 million and exports of £815 million. Traffic across the North Atlantic amounted to 253,000 tons, the equivalent of thirty general-cargo ships' voyages. This silent transfer goes on with little publicity. One shipper after another, urged on by labour stoppages, explores the chances of transferring his business to air. The loss of the products of the individual shipper may not be noticed by the port authority or by labour. There is the danger that new traffic may take to air as the normal transport. Particularly is this the case with electrical machinery, scientific, and professional instruments; of the latter category, 38 per cent went by air in 1966. BOAC profited considerably from the strike of United States dockers in December 1968.

All air terminals are investing in new transit buildings where cargo is controlled by computers and automated methods.[1]

In 1970 the Boeing 747, the Jumbo Jet, commenced a service from the United States to London where preparations are well advanced for handling the 110 tons of cargo each jet can carry.

Nationalization of Ports

The ambition that conditions in United Kingdom ports would be improved by worker participation finds expression in schemes for the nationalization of the industry or parts of it still in private or corporative hands. Many think that however important this aspect, the industry is not and will not be for some time, in a state to cope with so drastic a change. Containers, bulk cargoes, mechanization, and redundancy are problems that call for a period of calm adjustment and not revolutionary upheaval. Were it possible to take nationalization of ports out of politics and to judge it entirely from the standpoint of port efficiency, then a solution and a timing beneficial to the industry might be reached. Labour sees a chance to take part in port management. Employers argue against further upheaval, while admitting the case for a strong central controlling body, on the lines of the present National Ports Council. The need for research on a national scale is admitted; technical advance should be co-ordinated, and progress in standardization of equipment for ports could be possible.

The disadvantages of the present system arise entirely from the haphazard growth which has taken place in the United Kingdom since the Industrial Revolution of the eighteenth century. There are far too many ports, there is duplication of functions, fragmentation of responsibility for the daily work, and far too much documentation and paper chasing. Port authorities are too often in the dubious position of having responsibility without power.

Advocates of nationalization claim that one employer would make for better ship turnround. The stupendous changes that are shattering the accepted pattern of the industry can be tackled by a nationalized body which would command the co-operation of labour. There is not much in the history of the nationalized ports to support the argument that "them and us" would disappear on vesting day. It is true that the often poignant

---

[1] Airlines have now expanded their freight business to a point where they are having to invest in highly automated equipment at their freight terminals. They are also learning about that bane of all transport undertakings—the small parcel.

problems of redundancy could be handled more satisfactorily if the resources of the whole country could be called upon.

Like all schemes for nationalization, the first casualty is always the personal relations that have, for so many years, cemented the organization that is being replaced. The world in which ports operate is unlike that of any other industry. Until very recently the staff remained a tight and compact grouping, promotion from outside was rare, generations from the same family served the old dock companies and their successors, and, despite occupational grumbling, ports benefited from the intense loyalty of a staff to whom their job was their life work. It is claimed that all this was narrow and gave nothing but a practical outlook. Promotion and working conditions under nationalization would be determined not only on a regional but national basis, and the family feeling would disappear. Whilst competition would be abolished—that between the eight regions proposed under the scheme for nationalizing the ports of Great Britain would be too fictitious to be taken seriously—there would remain built-in anomalies within the proposed regions. The large disparity is quoted between the dues on ships imposed on the Medway; they are about one-sixth of those of the Port of London, which would be the controlling port of the proposed Thames and Medway region.

The surplus earned on its 1968 trading by British Transport Docks Board is posed against deficits in ports still under corporative control. This may make a good headline for the Press but it is unlikely to convince any port operator who has, in his early life, learnt that one can rarely compare like with like in an industry where no two ports are ever alike.

Perhaps the sanest conclusion that emerges from the welter of arguments is to leave the ports to convalesce after the major operation of the container and the bulk cargo before subjecting them to that of nationalization.

Additional Notes

Chapter 12, page 188, par. 2. Reduction in number of ships. Predicted by a London firm of shipping agents is a reduction of 847 conventional cargo carriers by 1973.

Page 198, par. 3. Nationalization of ports. A Bill to nationalize British ports was dropped with the change of government in Great Britain in June 1970.

Page 191, par. 1. Labour's reaction. Labour is beginning to appreciate the growing danger. A few London dockers at a training school passed a resolution drawing the attention of the employers to the situation.

Page 197, par. 3. Air freight. The national dock strike of July 1970 gave a fillip to air freight.

CHAPTER 13

THE LAST WORD

IN CONCLUDING this review of a rapidly changing transport industry one must face the fact that new systems and new requirements will eventually place both sea and air ports into the pattern of the future as nothing more than freight interchange stations between different transport methods. The concept of "through transport charges" has led exporters all over the world to consider how much is added to the cost of their goods in the market place by packaging and movement, storage and insurance, and interest on the capital tied up in products—moving or standing still— between the end of the production line and the handover to the final purchaser. *Every time a product is moved or handled something is added to the cost but nothing is added to the value.* With this truism in mind, the producer—faced with increasing market opportunities (as emergent or backward areas become more sophisticated) and increasing competition— will utilize every possible method to reduce those costs. In such circumstances the service-providers will have no alternative but to tailor their services to the requirements of the producers. It may happen that with improved methods of atmosphere control, fresh produce will no longer be dependent upon speed of movement. If it should prove cheaper to control the ripening processes of fruit in transit than to increase the handling and transit speeds, then the producers will demand the provision of atmosphere-controlled vehicles and will not use high-speed vehicles operating at high costs.

This is only one example. Where goods can be transported across a land mass more cheaply than they can be carried round a long coast line, then fast and cheap tranship methods will be demanded at the requisite points. And, eventually, someone will be able to provide that service and producers will use it. This is another example. The ultimate conclusion is that the cargo producers will dictate the kind of transport that will operate profitably. Technical advance will enable this to happen and so it will be.

Inevitably there will be less need for physical effort and a greater need for technicians. It is quite probable that even the geography of transport will change with aircraft capable of carrying loads that will make them fully intermodal with other forms of transport and freight submarines taking shorter routes under Arctic ice.

This kind of development cannot now be dismissed as science fiction. It is with such developments in mind that managements and staffs will eventually have to meet and decide what the future holds for them all. One thing that they *must* achieve will be efficiency, for whosoever fails to be efficient will soon be out of the race altogether. Port management and port workers will be no exception to requirements of reliability and efficiency. Industries will site themselves where they can gain the great advantage from trade routes which can supply their raw materials and along which they can reach their major markets. Such sites may or may not be on or near a coast or estuarial river. When they are not, then it will be useless for the ports to claim that work which could be more effectively or more cheaply carried out at an inland point is a traditional "port" operation.

The ultimate factor deciding the future transport problems may well be the abilities of city planners to design urban traffic facilities, because whatever ingenuity may be shown within the transport industry to bypass, fly over, or move under the larger conurbations, in the end the great majority of manufactured goods and fresh produce has to be delivered within the urban areas; and no part of a chain can be hauled indefinitely at a greater speed than the rest. Real efficiency will be achieved only by taking heed of all factors.

APPENDIX I

SUGGESTED ORGANIZATION OF A LIGHTERAGE DEPARTMENT TO BE RESPONSIBLE TO THE PORT AUTHORITY

STAFF REQUIRED

One officer-in-charge. He should have had practical experience of lighterage work and be capable of organizing and controlling labour.

One deputy. He should have similar qualifications and be capable of taking charge.

Two clerks. To keep records of work done, maintenance of craft, payment of wages, and general administration.

Six lightermen. A commencement should be made with this number. The number may be added to for extra work, holidays and sickness.

EQUIPMENT

Twelve barges. The flat-platformed type of dummy barge is suggested.

One tug, medium horse power; to be determined by weather and other conditions in the port.

Three mobile cranes and forklift trucks for the lighter berth. A supply of pallets.

INSTALLATION

A quay about 180 metres in length with good back storage and good surface. Good rail and road connections. An adequate ramp on which lorries can move from and to the quay and the deck of the pontoon.

MAINTENANCE

Small drydock for the maintenance of craft. Port engineers will look after the tug.

NOTE

The true function of a lighterage department must be appreciated. Lighterage is a transit operation for the purpose of reducing congestion on the quays, thereby turning ships round more quickly. Full barges must be discharged without delay to ensure a continuous movement of craft back to the ship. IN NO CIRCUMSTANCES MAY BARGES BE USED AS TEMPORARY WAREHOUSES. Palletized cargo can be loaded on to the deck of a barge by forklift truck.

APPENDIX II

SUGGESTED ORGANIZATION OF A RAILWAY DEPARTMENT BY A PORT AUTHORITY

THE best results can be obtained by the port authority assuming responsibility for rail traffic from a point at the exit to the marshalling yard and
retaining it until the wagons are handed over at this, or another point to
be agreed, after completion of their use within the port area. The advantages of this assumption of responsibility by the port authority have been
proved over the years.

(1) The port operator has control over the number of wagons he needs
    for his daily work.
(2) He can give orders to and get them carried out by staff working
    for the same employer.
(3) Shunting to his requirements can be done quickly by using tractors
    independently of the state railways.
(4) Possession of a minimum number of shunting engines by the port
    authority renders them independent of the state railway who do
    not always give priority to the needs of the docks.
(5) It should be the general aim of a port authority to assume more and
    more responsibility for the operations that take place within the
    dock estate. Divided responsibility is the enemy of efficiency.

STAFF REQUIRED

One railway superintendent, experienced in rail working and able to
work in harmony with the state railway officials.

One deputy superintendent, prepared to act in the absence of his
principal.

Two railway inspectors to supervise daily working.

Two clerks to administer the department and to keep records.

Six shunters and tractor drivers.

EQUIPMENT

Shunting engines and tractors with normal rail equipment as necessary. The system should be run on common sense lines with no signalling.

ADMINISTRATION

A small office in or near the marshalling yard is necessary.

INDEX